**This book is to be returned on or before
the last date stamped below.**

ROBERTS

Severe Accidental Head Injury

Severe Accidental Head Injury

An Assessment of Long-term Prognosis

A. H. Roberts

First published 1979 by
THE MACMILLAN PRESS LTD
London and Basingstoke
Associated companies in Delhi Dublin
Hong Kong Johannesburg Lagos Melbourne
New York Singapore and Tokyo

Filmset by VANTAGE PHOTOSETTING CO. LTD.
Southampton and London
Printed in Great Britain by
UNWIN BROTHERS LTD
The Gresham Press, Old Woking, Surrey

British Library Cataloguing in Publication Data

Roberts, Anthony Herber
  Severe accidental head injury.
  1. Head – Wounds and injuries
  I. Title
  617'.1   RD521

  ISBN 0–333–27015–0

Foreword

Walpole Lewin CBE, DSc, MS, FRCS
Consultant Neurological Surgeon, Addenbrookes Hospital, Cambridge

This book is published at a most opportune time for those concerned in the study of head injuries. There have been significant advances in recent years, not only in our understanding of the underlying physiological and pathological changes that may follow injury, but also in management. They include the demonstration of the pathology of concussion; the use of controlled ventilation to prevent hypoxia and to assist in the maintenance of normal intracranial pressure; the introduction of computerised axial tomography as a non-invasive examination in the diagnosis of some complicating factors after head injury, particularly intracranial haematoma; the recognition of the metabolic and hormonal changes that may follow severe brain injury. These and other factors have placed into the hands of doctors valuable adjuncts to the diagnosis of head injury and the prevention and management of potentially fatal complications.

The questions being asked now, however, concern not only what effect these changes have on the mortality rate, but after severe head injury what is the quality of life for those who survive? Can we predict what is likely to happen at various intervals following injury, and what measures are required to mitigate the long-term effects among the survivors?

One approach to answering these questions is provided in this book based on a meticulous study of a series of consecutive head injuries followed up for periods from ten to twenty-five years. The survey was conducted, not by those concerned in the acute management, but by an independent team headed by Dr Anthony Roberts, Consultant Neurologist in London, and assisted by Mrs Dorothy Weir, Psychiatric Social Worker, and Dr Eileen Smith, Clinical Psychologist. It says much for their dedication that of the 548 patients studied, all but 11 were traced after such long periods of time.

In this book the reader will find some useful prognostic factors which should help him in trying to answer some of the difficult questions doctors ask themselves, as do the patients and their relatives. The survey graphically demonstrates the practical recovery many patients can make, especially the young; but it also emphasises in poignant fashion the problems and difficulties a family may face when one of their number is left with major mental and/or physical disability. The challenge to doctors from the evidence provided is the implication that the ultimate result may depend not only on the severity of the initial injuries, but on the treatment given in the immediate period afterwards when time is of the essence and when some complications can be prevented and others treated before irreversible changes take place.

The closing chapters of this book emphasise the rising tide of patients, mainly young people, left either totally dependent on others or severely disabled. Is society fully aware of the need to make adequate provision for their care, and will the evidence stimulate us to re-examine our rehabilitation programmes and to attend to the mental needs of patients and their relatives with as much energy that some expend on purely physical rehabilitation?

I am personally very grateful to Dr Roberts for undertaking this research and for providing for all of us concerned in the management of head injuries much that will be useful in the care of patients, and pointers to some of the changes that are so urgently required in the future if we are to raise our standards of care.

Contents

Foreword by Mr Walpole Lewin   v

Acknowledgements   viii

1 Introduction   1

2 Previous Reports of Long-term Outcome   4

3 Method of Patient Selection and Design of the Investigation   22

4 The Patients and their Injuries   29

5 Patterns of Residual Central Neural Lesions and Associated Disabilities   39

6 Patterns of Personality Disorder and Intellectual and Memory Deficits   55

7 Cranial Nerve Injuries, Vertigo and Headache   89

8 Pituitary and Hypothalamic Disorders   102

9 Systemic Complications and Peripheral Nerve, Bone and Joint Injury   111

10 Prevalence and Natural History of Post-traumatic Epilepsy   118

11 Progressive Post-traumatic Encephalopathy and Premature Ageing   129

12 Life Expectancy and Causes of Death   140

13 Predicting the Long-term Outcome   152

14 Summary, Conclusions and Implications   180

Appendix: Illustrative Cases   191

References   207

Index   220

Acknowledgements

I am indebted to Mr J. C. Scott, Mr J. B. Pennybacker and Mr Walpole Lewin, formerly of the Accident and Neurosurgical Services at the Radcliffe Infirmary, Oxford, for permission to examine those patients previously under their care; to Mr Walpole Lewin and Mr John Potter and their colleagues, whose detailed documentation of the original case histories made this study possible; to Mr T. F. de C. Marshall of the Department of Medical Statistics and Epidemiology at the London School of Hygiene and Tropical Medicine, for his computer-assisted analysis of the results and his invaluable help on the epidemiological aspects of this study; to Dr B. Baughan of the Institute of Education Computing Centre, London, who wrote the computer programme for and gave advice on the statistical analysis of Dr Eileen Smith's psychometric assessments; and to Dr F. Newcombe for her advice on the selection of the most suitable psychometric tests.

I am very greatly indebted to Dr Eileen Smith, Senior Clinical Psychologist at the National Hospitals for Nervous Diseases, London, for her valuable contribution to this study; to Mrs D. M. Weir, Psychiatric Social Worker for her assistance; and to Miss M. Hargreaves for tracing many of the patients by house to house enquiries.

The task of tracing would not have been practicable without the assistance of the staff of the General Register Office, in particular Mr D. J. Smale and many of his colleagues.

The survey was financed by a research grant from the Department of Health and Social Security.

In Miss Kathleen Dyer I have had the good fortune to have had helping me, in two epidemiological studies of head injury, a former nursing sister, medical librarian and bibliographer equipped with a first class degree in modern languages. It is a pleasure to acknowledge my very considerable debt to her and my gratitude.

I am very grateful to Dr Ronald Henson for his continued encouragement, and to Professors Bryan Jennett and Alwyn Lishman for their critical comments.

1 Introduction

The past 30 years has seen, in most developed countries, a steady increase in the proportion of the population who can expect to suffer head injury. At the same time, improvements in techniques of resuscitation and in the management and effective treatment of some of the complications of head injury have salvaged a progressively larger number of the more severely brain-damaged who would previously have had no chance of surviving their injury.

The greater proportion of those involved in accidents which cause head injury are healthy adolescents and young adults who, at the time of the injury, have a further life expectancy of a half century or more in the normal course of events. There must therefore be a substantial and steadily enlarging population of more or less disabled survivors of head injury making increasing demands on the societies in which they live. Despite this there is still surprisingly little information about this important and almost certainly underprivileged minority group within the community.

The published facts do not provide a clear idea to what extent the various disabilities characteristic of brain damage due to closed head injury may be expected to resolve or become modified in the long term, or how often and in what form they are likely to persist indefinitely. There is little information about the ultimate prospects for the more severely disabled and less on life expectancy. What there is tends to be conflicting since it has usually been based on heterogeneous series of patients selected by criteria which are difficult to compare and often poorly defined.

It is generally held that as much recovery of function as is going to take place after brain tissue has been destroyed is likely to have done so in the course of a year or so. It is a common observation that the rate of recovery of function after brain injury declines exponentially with time, but to determine at what stage it ceases, or when it can be assumed that no further modification of disordered function can be expected, requires the assessment of residual disability in an unbiased sample from an unselected population of head-injured patients followed over many years.

In addition, any assessment of post-traumatic neural disability must attempt a separate examination of the contributions to the overall incapacity made by impaired memory and other intellectual functions, and by personality disorder, as well as by physical disability. Such information is available in some detail in a number of studies of war wounded, but this kind of population is highly contaminated by patients with penetrating brain wounds due to small, high-velocity missiles. The damage caused by these missiles is unlike the diffuse acceleration injury to the brain which occurs in the more common closed head injuries of accidents. Studies of the long-term disabilities of wartime brain injury may relate to those of closed head injury caused by accidents, but this can only be decided when comparable data are available from both sources.

The prospect of analysing in great detail functional disturbances caused by the discrete focal brain injury of high-velocity missiles has encouraged a number of exceptionally well-designed studies of this type of head injury in relation to traumatic personality disorder, impaired intellectual function and memory, as well as in the coarser field of disordered sensory perception, motor function and epilepsy. There have been few attempts to define patterns of disordered neural function after closed head injury, and even fewer designed to examine the relationship between disabilities still demonstrable many years afterwards and the individual characteristics of the head injury. This has been so despite the theoretical, experimental and pathological evidence that the brain damage in closed head injury, although diffuse, is usually most severe in polar and medial temporal and orbitofrontal areas of the brain, and that there is a predictable relationship to the site of head impact.

In a study of the cumulative effects of repeated minor head injuries in a random selection of boxers examined many years after the end of their professional careers, the author noted a relatively stereotyped clinical syndrome. This suggested damage preferentially to areas of the brain concerned with memory, together with an asymmetrical distribution of the intensity of the injury in cerebellar and pyramidal systems. A striking feature of this pattern of lesions was the frequency with which signs of pyramidal damage were more marked in the left limbs. This observation, which was also seen to have been made by others when earlier reports of boxers' encephalopathy were analysed in detail, is undoubtedly related to the fact that in boxing there is a tendency for more and harder blows to be struck by the right fist to the left side of the head. It seemed likely that if this were apparent after repeated minor head injury, there may be a more accurately predictable relationship in severe closed head injury between the side of head impact and post-traumatic disorders of intellectual function and perhaps of personality, as well as weakness and ataxia of the limbs.

The undeniable disadvantages of retrospective studies are lessened when the aim is the assessment of the ultimate outlook for disabilities which result from severe head injury. Questions of prediction which concern the surgeon in his management of the patient in the first hours or days after head injury are not the same as those posed for the physician who is attempting, several weeks or months later, to assess the most opportune time to introduce the available techniques of physical or mental, and finally social and occupational, rehabilitation. And they hardly concern those advising on the problem of appropriate financial compensation for disabilities likely to persist. In viewing the natural history of the effects of brain damage in head injury it is easier to see the evolution of a pattern of disability if the information about the acute and convalescent stages can be compared with the state of the patient examined years later, shorn of the distracting problems of acute management.

The study described in this monograph was designed to examine the relationship between the type and severity of non-missile head injury and early neurological sequelae, and the final degree and characteristics of mental and physical disability between 3 and 25 years later in two groups of patients. The first, a consecutive series, included every patient remaining unconscious or amnestic for a week or longer from a total population of 7000 patients admitted after head injury to the Accident Service of the Radcliffe Infirmary, Oxford between 1948 and 1961. This was for practical purposes a random sample, and estimates based on these figures are made for the numbers similarly disabled after head injury annually in England and Wales in the final chapter. To these patients were added a smaller selected series of the most severely head injured, drawn from other sources, who had remained unconscious for longer than a month after injury.

Details of the acute and convalescent stages after injury were abstracted from the uniformly well-documented case records of neurosurgical units with a particular interest in the management of head injuries. Of the total series of 548 patients only 11 were lost to the survey and the rest were followed up and re-examined, or the cause and time of death were established. In each case the persisting intellectual, personality and neural deficits found, and the disabilities these caused in the spheres of domestic social and occupational life were assessed. In nearly 90 per cent of cases a similarly detailed account was obtained from one or more relatives. The majority were also examined by a neuropsychologist using tests of intellectual function designed to demonstrate memory and intellectual functional deficits lateralised to one or other cerebral hemisphere.

A computer-assisted analysis of the data made it possible to describe patterns of residual neural lesions, often predictably related to the severity and complications of the injury and to the side of head impact in the less severely injured, and to suggest probable pathological correlations; to predict, in most cases within weeks of injury, the final degree and character of personality disorder, intellectual deficit and neural disability to be expected in the long term, and the rate at which recovery is likely to take place; to make estimates of life expectancy and examine the natural history of post-traumatic epilepsy; and to deny the entity of a specific neuronal degeneration due to a single head injury. Each of these topics is considered separately, as the titles of the chapters indicate, and discussed in the light of earlier studies. They follow a review of previous publications on the general subject of long-term prognosis after severe closed head injury, and in the appendix there are examples of case records illustrating the patterns of mental and physical disability that were found.

2 Previous Reports of Long-term Outcome

This chapter provides a critical survey of those previous reports in which the design of the investigation and methods of assessment were sufficiently clearly described to make possible comparisons with the present study. There is also a voluminous literature on the general topic of the neurology, pathology and mechanics of closed head injury to which reference is made in the relevant chapters.

Unfortunately, methods of assessment and criteria for the selection of patients, and even the interpretation of 'long-term' and 'severe', vary so widely in these reports that it is impossible to present all the information adequately in tabular form alone: more extended discussion is necessary. The following account comments on similarities and differences, and also on inadequacies or limitations of method or selection criteria, whilst at the same time drawing attention to the numbers of patients studied on which conclusions have been based.

The reports are reviewed in order of their comparability with the present study, the most closely comparable first. There is further subdivision into three sections reflecting the selection criteria employed in each case. The first section deals with those papers in which the severity of the injury has been estimated indirectly by the duration of coma or post-traumatic amnesia, or by the characteristics of the neurological state during the acute traumatic period. The second reviews papers in which the selection of patients has been made on the basis of the severity of physical disability requiring physiotherapeutic rehabilitation in convalescence. In the third section age has been the primary criterion for selection, and those reports are reviewed which are concerned with the long-term outcome of severe closed head injury in children. Finally, brief reference is made to a few studies which, although reporting only the short-term outcome, examine issues highly relevant to the general problem of prediction.

Selection of Patients by Criteria of Severity of Injury

The most closely comparable study, so far as attempts to examine individually the various disabling sequelae are concerned, is that reported by Fahy, Irving and Millac (1967). In this a rather idiosyncratic criterion of severity was used for the selection of the patients. This was that the state of the patient on admission to hospital had been such as to indicate the need for burr-hole exploration. This was normally done in any patient in coma who did not 'show and sustain signs of improvement within a short time of admission'. Sixty-seven consecutively injured patients were selected, excluding cases with depressed skull fractures, and also three patients who, in retrospect, were thought to have had injuries insufficiently severe to warrant the surgical exploration to which they had been submitted. The 32 survivors were traced 6 years after their injury. The cause of death for the six who were found to have died was established and all but two of the remaining 26 who were still alive were personally examined by the authors. There is no comment as to the duration of coma, but the post-traumatic amnesia had exceeded 3 days in all cases, the mean post-traumatic amnesia being 5 weeks. The brain had been seen to be contused or lacerated in nearly half the cases and there was surface brain compression in more than a third.

In assessing the outcome the authors considered neurological disability, psychiatric aspects, post-concussional symptoms, epilepsy and work capacity separately. It was found that a third of the patients were without neurological signs, and that recovery from hemiparesis or bilateral spasticity was good, so that in the five patients with persisting hemiparesis disability was slight and the majority had only residual changes in tendon reflexes and plantar responses. A disturbance of gait, due in a third of the cases to cerebellar damage, and in two patients to spasticity of the legs, was mild. A sensory deficit was demonstrable in only two cases and it was limited to patchy impairment of perception of pain. The most severe neurological disability was due not to central neural damage, but to a peripheral brachial plexus lesion. Complaints of speech disturbance were apparently frequent, but it is not clear whether in most instances this was due to a defect of articulation rather than dysphasia. One patient still had a mild naming difficulty. Residual cranial nerve lesions were limited to a complete loss of sense of smell in three instances, unilateral optic nerve damage in three others and mild oculomotor impairment in two.

So far as psychiatric sequelae were concerned less than a quarter of those examined were judged to the symptom-free, and half were demented, assessed by tests of intellectual function. The remaining quarter were forgetful but not sufficiently so for this to be demonstrable in psychometric tests of memory. A schizophreniform psychosis developed in one demented patient, and two of the forgetful ones had paranoid delusional illnesses. In others disinhibition, moods of depression and a variety of 'angry and depressive feelings' were said to be in contrast to their previous personalities. One patient became prone to outbursts of violence and another was considered to have become introverted and obsessional. There were two patients who were considered to have undergone welcome changes in personality as a result of their injuries. Impaired concentration and increased irritability were common, but the association of these two symptoms with complaints of headache, giddiness and intolerance of noise, as is characteristic of the so-called post-concussional syndrome, was not encountered.

It was shown that there was increasing neurological and psychiatric disability with longer post-traumatic amnesia, and that psychiatric disability was greater than neurological. Neither was severe when the amnesia had lasted for only 2 weeks. Half of those whose post-traumatic amnesia had lasted for 7 weeks were left with severe disabilities in both spheres. No significant relationships were found between neuropsychiatric disability and age, or duration of coma, although no statement was made as to the period of coma the patients had experienced. All informants reported that disabilities improved during the first 2 years, this improvement still continuing in a third of the patients at 4 years. The mortality rate amongst the survivors discharged from hospital was six times that expected in a normal population of similar age, and half of these had died severely demented in mental hospitals. A fifth of the survivors were unemployed at the time of the examination but half of the remainder were earning as much as before injury. Full employment with some reduction in earning capacity was possible despite quite severe physical disability. Objective measures of social adjustment seemed to bear little relation to clinical findings. It was not apparent to the authors how the outcome 6 years later might have been predicted on the information available in the year of the injury.

A number of other studies have been reported in the last 10 years in which the design and methods of investigation have been similar but, because there has been selection bias, the information derived from them is open to more criticism. Miller and Stern (1965) selected 100 consecutive patients, who had been referred to one of them, on average 3 years after injury, for medical assessment in connection with claims for compensation. Ninety-two survivors were then re-examined between 3 and 40 years later. In each case the post-traumatic amnesia had lasted for more than 24 hours. It was found that, of the four who had died in the interval, in only one case was death related to the head injury. This had been due to poisoning by coal gas which the patient could not smell. Residual psychiatric symptoms were present in about 15 per cent. Rather more than half of these showed some degree of dementia. A further four patients were to some extent disabled by neurotic anxiety and depression, two being constitutionally predisposed. Evidence of focal brain injury, demonstrable at the first examination in a quarter of the series as a spastic weakness on one or both sides was found persisting in only four patients at the time of the follow-up studies. Limb ataxia persisted in only one, and hemisensory loss in none. No patient had residual dysphasia. Impairment of cranial nerve function was still evident in most cases where the first, second and eighth nerves were involved, although to what extent and what disability this caused is not mentioned. Post-traumatic epilepsy developed in almost a fifth of these patients and most remained liable to fits. Three were still having frequent attacks despite anticonvulsant medication. The occupational status of a quarter of the men had declined as a result of their injury, about a third of these because of permanent brain damage, and in the majority of the rest as a result of 'impairment of efficiency' not otherwise specified. Epilepsy was contributory to this downgrading in six patients. All the children had recovered completely and all the women seemed to have been capable of looking after their homes, although how efficiently is not stated. These authors do not comment on factors affecting prognosis amongst their patients.

In a more recent paper, Lundholm, Jepsen and Thornval (1975) selected a consecutive series of 54 patients who had been unconscious for more than a week after injury, and re-examined the 30 survivors between 8 and 14 years later. There were three injuries complicated by surface brain compression; the remaining patients were considered to have suffered cerebral contusion. Their social rehabilitation was graded as independent, dependent in some degree upon their families or an institution but able to take care of their personal needs, or helpless and requiring permanent institutional care. The grade of rehabilitation was examined in relation to persisting neurological and intellectual functional impairment. Varying degrees of paresis persisted in all three groups, but no more severely amongst those who were completely dependent than amongst those who were not. On the other hand amongst the quarter of the patients with severe mental impairment none was socially independent; half were independent but only one of these was over the age of forty at the time of his injury. The length of coma within each age group was another determinant of outcome. Coma exceeding a month precluded rehabilitation if the injury occurred over the age of twenty. It was considered that all of the patients exhibited some intellectual impairment, and two-thirds 'an abnormal behaviour pattern' not otherwise qualified.

A small number of patients whose head injuries had caused coma lasting for at least 3 weeks were followed up by van der Zwan (1969). In this report he reviews the same series of patients followed for a shorter time 5 years earlier and described in greater detail by Lambooy, van der Zwan and Fossen (1965). In defining their concept of grades of coma they assess as conscious patients who were 'following with the eyes' and note that of the 14 unconscious for longer than 2 months, half died, whilst all the survivors remained 'severely disabled'. Of the 44 patients selected, more than a third were either dead or not available for examination, but the remaining 27 patients were examined personally by the authors. In a quarter of these surface compression by intercranial bleeding had complicated the injury and a tracheostomy had been required in nearly every case. Neurological abnormalities due to central lesions caused a persisting hemi- or monoparesis in a third of the patients and in two cases these were still severely disabling. A third of the cases were affected by incoordination and in half of these there was a paresis of the legs. Akinesia tended to be more disabling than paralysis. In half the patients speech was a flat monotone. There was little demonstrable sensory loss, but what there was tended to be associated with severe hemiparesis. Evidence of disturbed endocrine function was present in only one case and this solely on account of obesity. There was persisting anosmia, or an optic nerve lesion, in over a third, and residual facial paralysis in another third. Eighth nerve function remained impaired in nearly half. In all the patients there was a marked slowness of thought, speech and movement which varied in degree. Tests of memory were impaired in two-thirds, and a third were to some extent dysphasic. In general the prevalence of residual disabilities due to central neural lesions doubled where the coma lasted for longer than a month. This was not found to be so in the case of intellectual impairment assessed by psychometric tests, nor in the case of behaviour disorders. These latter were reminiscent of the effects of standard leucotomies. A quarter were socially dependent, another quarter were able to earn a living but at a reduced level, and the remaining patients had not changed their social status.

In a large number of reports of the long-term outcome the period of follow-up has ranged extensively from a few months to several years and the value of the assessments is for this reason open to criticism. A careful clinical study was made by Frowein, Haar, Terhaag, Kinzel and Wieck (1968) based on a consecutive series of 132 patients who had been unconscious for longer than 2 days. Unconsciousness, precisely defined, was considered to last until the patient kept his eyes open in response to painful stimuli or command, or until he carried out specific movements on command. One quarter of the patients were lost to the survey and the remaining 100 were followed up between 1 and 13 years later, half for no more than 6 years. Residual neurological disability consisting of severe paresis was present in a quarter of all the patients followed up, and slight pareses were present in another tenth. Where this type of neural disability was severe it was associated with considerable limitation in work capacity. Slight paralyses recovered within 6 months, and increasingly longer periods were needed before the final level of improvement was reached in the more severe forms. In some children improvement continued for 5 years. The striking improvement in spastic paresis commented on by Miller and Stern (1965) was observed in only one case. In adults paresis could take 3 years to recover, but there was rarely significant improvement thereafter.

A series of tests held to assess various aspects of intellectual and personality deterioration, as designed by Kinzel (1968), was used in a random sample of 38 per cent of the patients studied by Frowein *et al.* It would appear from the authors' diagrams that, overall, there was a positive correlation between low test scores and poor occupational rehabilitation. To a lesser extent there was the same relationship with duration of coma. The euphoria exhibited by many of the severely damaged patients often tended to be misleading in the assessment of outcome. An analysis was made of the relationship between duration of coma and capacity for work. It was concluded that, for children, normal or only slightly limited working capacity would follow coma prolonged for 3 weeks, but for adults up to the age of forty-five years 1 week was the limit, and for those older, no more than 4 days. In only a quarter of the patients, of whom over half were under the age of twenty, was the working capacity judged to be normal, and in severe cases it took as long as 4 years to reach this level of rehabilitation. In the case of the more severely damaged patients rehabilitation in some kind of sheltered employment was not achieved until 9 years after the injury.

In a consecutive series of 308 patients who had suffered what is described as 'severe cerebral injuries' with and without fracture of the skull, Sölch and Schyra (1972) examined the relationship between the duration of unconsciousness, three grades of severity of the injury and the outcome 2–20 years later. Severity was assessed by considering the time needed for the initial neurological defect to regress. Those who regained their mobility early on had fewer neurological signs when followed up. It is not clear what proportion of the survivors were followed up or how many were personally examined. They noted, as have preceding authors, that three-quarters of the patients could be considered to have recovered from their injury and that disability in the remainder was due mainly to personality change, intellectual deficits and epilepsy. Most of the patients under the age of twenty years regained their capacity to work, and proportionately larger numbers failed to do this as age increased. The duration of coma, not otherwise defined, similarly affected occupational status. Unconsciousness persisting 3 days and more resulted in some limitation of the capacity to work normally in the majority. Dementia was rare and massive cerebral deficits were seldom seen. On the other hand, what they describe as 'micro-symptoms', which include clinical signs of pyramidal tract lesions, were common and still present in over a third when re-examined. Fewer than a tenth had actual paresis of a limb. The intellectual and psychiatric symptoms were the most severe consequences of the injury which persisted. The most striking was a general slowing down of thought processes with defects of day-to-day memory, loss of initiative and irritability. This was noted in about a fifth of the cases. Severe frontal personality change was present, with some degree of dementia, in about a tenth of their patients. The authors review the evidence which suggests that many of these sequelae are due, not to primary traumatic brain damage, but to a number of interacting factors such as predisposition, raised intracranial pressure and secondary lesions.

Selecting on the basis of coma lasting for longer than a month, Lecuire, Deruty, Dechaume and Lapras (1973) followed 37 survivors of 69 patients for a period of over 18 months. The authors did not define precisely their concept of coma but they note that most of their patients required tracheostomy and many needed assisted respiration. They observe in general terms that both age and length of coma determine prognosis. Despite neurological deficits the larger proportion of their patients was able to take up paid work again. Disorders of personality and intellectual function typically included impairment of memory and concentration and of the ability to make sustained intellectual effort. This was usually associated with irritability, aggression and emotional instability. This characteristic constellation of disordered mentality frequently 'compromised rehabilitation' even when neurological and intellectual functions were otherwise relatively unimpaired.

A study of 100 consecutive patients who had suffered a head injury defined as severe, in that they had been unable to answer or obey for longer than 9 days, was reported by Obrador, Bustos and Fernandez-Ruiz (1973). They were re-examined between 8 months and 7 years later. Rather less than a third had undergone surgical removal of contused or lacerated temporal or frontal poles, or evacuation of compressive surface collections of blood or fluid. A close relationship was shown to exist between the length of post-traumatic amnesia and the duration of unconsciousness, or what the authors prefer to describe in terms of varying grades of 'subreactivity'. Three-quarters were found to have some degree of major neurological deficit. This was severe in less than a tenth, and a quarter also had sensory defects. A third were dysphasic in some degree and two-thirds had defective 'recent memory'. It was the authors' impression that the likelihood of further recovery of neural function after 3 years was remote. Increasing age, duration of post-traumatic amnesia and the duration of 'subreactivity', that is, impaired response to stimulation after the injury, was associated with an increasing prevalence of intellectual defects as tested, and with a decline in occupational status. Substantially less than a quarter had returned to their former occupations at the time they were followed up, but there is no comment on how long this was in each case. A return to some form of work was usual in patients below the age of forty whose post-traumatic amnesia had lasted for less than 40 days. No patient over the age of forty at the time of injury was able to work normally again. In most cases recovery sufficient to enable the patient to return to work had taken place within a year – if it were going to.

Selection by Criteria of Severity of Persisting Physical Disability in Convalescence

In all the previous reports selection has been by an indirect criterion of severity of the injury based upon the duration of traumatic amnesia, coma or altered consciousness, or, in the first paper, by a somewhat less easily comparable assessment of the need for burr-hole exploration because of deterioration or lack of improvement in conscious level and neural responsiveness.

A well-documented study of 170 patients selected from amongst 617 who still had severe disabilities at the time of discharge from hospital or several months later, was reported by Vigouroux, Baurand, Choux and Guillermain (1972). These were followed up between 1 and 12 years later. Over half of the patients did not reply to the appeal to collaborate, and of the 352 who did, it would seem, although this is nowhere clearly stated, that all were examined personally by the authors. The 182 they judged to be almost normal were excluded from the study. Case reports of the 14 individuals most seriously disabled, survivors of modern methods of resuscitation, are given in detail. Amongst these there were three whose neurological state is described as 'végétative', one being still alive 11 years after injury. There were two able to make semipurposive movement of a limb whose level of consciousness was such as to suggest some contact with their environment, but it is doubtful whether these were more than primitive automatisms.

The authors describe in some detail the characteristics of disordered motor function, cranial nerve deficits, and clinically demonstrable defects of intellectual function which they found amongst the remaining 156 patients. In only five of the 47 patients with residual pyramidal lesions were these considered to be severe; the degree of spasticity varied and most looked cortical in origin. There were 10 cases of extrapyramidal rest tremors and rigidity, most marked in an arm. They considered cerebellar ataxia and intention tremor to be rare, and identifiable in only seven cases. In an assessment of residual cranial nerve deficits the authors describe 13 patients who had unilateral optic atrophy, eight of these due either to a direct optic lesion or fracture of the base of the skull. One patient had bilateral optic atrophy and four patients had homonymous hemianopic field defects. The commonest oculomotor palsy seen was the third, of which there were nine cases. There was only one patient with a residual sixth nerve palsy, although two others had partial involvement of both third and sixth nerves. Residual facial paralysis due to seventh nerve lesions was found in 22 patients. Surprisingly, there were only five cases of complete anosmia. Deafness was found in 13 cases and labyrinthine function was seriously impaired in four cases.

In describing their clinical assessment of intellectual functions under the heading of 'disordered symbolic functions' they note 23 patients with some residual dysphasia, one with dyslexia and seven stutterers. They also mention here 12 additional patients with severe dysarthria. Another 21 patients were apraxic. No attempt is made in any of the foregoing to relate the various sequelae to the type of injury or to indices of severity available at, or shortly after the injury, which would enable predictions to be made. There was one case of extreme post-traumatic obesity which, together with a small number of other rare sequelae of severe head injury, they found difficult to classify. In their review of 'psychic and intellectual' sequelae they make the pertinent comment that every author uses his own personal nomenclature, thus making comparisons difficult. They themselves distinguish between four conditions. The first they describe as deficits of intellectual function which may be either transitory or permanent; the second, genuine post-traumatic neurosis; the third, various conditions which they describe as 'neuropathic', amongst which are included neurasthenia and hypochondriasis, simulated physical disabilities, phobias and a variety of paranoid attitudes and behaviour considered to be largely constitutionally predetermined; and the fourth, psychoses and dementia. In this latter group they noted two cases of schizophrenia but doubted the relevance of trauma in either, five cases of manic-depressive illness, and six cases of dementia for which they held the injury responsible.

In attempting to assess the outcome in terms of physical and social disability the authors make the point that it is often the interaction of various sequelae of the injury that disables, and they draw attention to the frequent association of disabling orthopaedic complications, in particular of what they describe as 'para-osteo-arthropathy'. Taking into account all these combined disabilities, there were three categories of outcome. The first comprised 104 'handicapped' patients, who had been rendered 'inferior' as a result of sequelae; there were 33 patients classified as 'infirmes', in whom one or several neural or orthopaedic functions were definitely 'altered'; and 19 patients termed '*invalides*' who were unable to work as a result of their disabilities. Case reports are given to illustrate the characteristics of each of these three categories, but no attempt is made to relate the outcome to indices of severity of the injury.

In a separate consideration of 53 patients selected from the 170 because they had survived coma lasting for 3 weeks or more, there is a careful analysis of the manner in which the length and grade of coma has determined outcome. A comparison was made between these patients and the 42 who had been excluded from the previous study because, when re-examined at the time of follow-up, they were considered to have no disabilities at all. The authors found a consistent relationship between increasing disability and the duration of coma and the grade of coma, defined on the basis of the character of the response to stimulation. Of those who were in coma from 3 weeks to 2 months, 55 per cent were considered to be left with no disability at all, 23 per cent to be handicapped, and the remaining 22 per cent to be disabled either socially or physically to a degree that made them dependent. The trends were reversed with coma lasting for 2 months in that only 12 per cent were considered free of disabilities, 4 per cent handicapped, but 84 per cent socially or physically dependent. Surprisingly, one patient, unconscious for longer than 3 months, was found to have no disabilities at all.

In the same way, of those patients whose grade of coma included decerebrate responses to stimulation, 28 per cent were left without disabling sequelae of any kind, 25 per cent were handicapped to some degree, and 47 per cent were dependent. Conversely, where the coma did not involve decerebration, 61 per cent were left without disabling sequelae, 11 per cent were handicapped and 28 per cent were disabled and dependent.

The most serious limitation of this study, which otherwise, of all the others reviewed here, approximates most closely in scale to the present investigation, is the failure to indicate in what proportion of patients the assessments were actually of the long- rather than the short-term outcome. Since time is so important a determinant of final outcome, this would seem a substantial drawback to the interpretation of the significance of many of their findings.

In a number of studies reported from rehabilitation units, admission to the unit has been the only criterion for selection. It is seldom apparent how the severity of the injuries originally sustained by the patients are to be otherwise classified and related to their final disabilities. Rusk, Block and Lowman (1969) re-examined a series of 118 patients 5–15 years after admission to their rehabilitation unit. The patients had suffered 'semiconsciousness, semicoma or coma', not otherwise qualified, which, on average, had lasted for 6 weeks after injury. The authors had excluded from their study a substantial number of patients who were decerebrate or otherwise too disabled for rehabilitation. In about a third the injury had been complicated by surface brain compression which had been treated surgically. After assessment in the unit rather less than a quarter were judged to be incapable of rehabilitation and, when followed up, these were found not to have improved. By the time of their discharge from the unit over half were either completely or partially independent and they were found to have maintained this level without any notable improvement. A small number who were just ambulant without assistance, or able to feed themselves without help by the time they left the unit, were subsequently found to have regressed. It was felt that this had been due to the inordinate effort needed to contend, amongst other difficulties, with the profound slowness of movement caused by their disabilities. No details are given, but it appears that after discharge from the unit there was often a tendency for neural disabilities increasingly to limit activities rather than for continuing improvement to take place. It is a measure of the extreme severity of the neural disabilities amongst these head-injured patients that in less than a fifth was ambulation 'unlimited', even at the time they left the unit.

A somewhat similar general review of 30 patients admitted to a rehabilitation unit in the U.K. was reported by Panting and Merry (1972). Coma, not otherwise defined, was taken as the index of severity and had extended for longer than a week in two-thirds of the cases. No attempt was made to examine further any relationship between length of coma and long-term disability. Just over half the patients were examined personally by the authors between 1 and 6 years after injury. It seemed that although residual pyramidal signs were commonly present they seldom led to any demonstrable loss of function, unlike the disabilities due to cerebellar incoordination and imbalance, which persisted in two-thirds of the cases. Visual field defects were responsible for the greatest disability in a few instances. It was found that these physical disabilities did not cause as much distress as personality disorder. The most striking and frequently encountered feature of this was violent and uncontrollable outbursts of rage. In some cases these were so explosive as to raise the possibility of epilepsy. Such irritability was seldom typical of their previous personalities, most having been stable. This severe disturbance of emotional control improved as recovery progressed. A third of the patients developed post-traumatic epilepsy, but in the majority the fits were relatively easy to control and the frequency of the attacks decreased.

Another brief report on 93 patients treated at a rehabilitation unit and followed up for 3 years or more was given by Bruckner and Randle (1972). Only two-thirds of the patients were re-examined by one of the authors. The criterion of severity for inclusion in the survey was post-traumatic amnesia of 24 hours or more and/or compound fracture of the skull or intracranial haemorrhage. A third of the patients failed to return to work.

The authors found that 'psychological symptoms' produced the most serious disabilities. These were present in two-thirds of the unemployed, compared with a tenth in those working at the same socioeconomic level as they had been prior to injury. In contrast to some of the previous reports the authors considered that a persistent hemiplegia did contribute to the failure to return to work in about tenth of the patients. Major factors adversely affecting return to work were age over forty years at the time of injury, impairment of memory, concentration and other intellectual functions, personality change, particularly that associated with aggression and causing depression, and loss of initiative. No attempt was made to assess in detail the relationship between the severity of the injury and the long-term outcome.

A more detailed assessment was made by Maury, Audic, Lacombe and Lucet (1970), although here it is unclear at what stage up to 7 years after their injuries each of the 94 patients was examined. In this series of patients selection for study was by admission to a rehabilitation unit, and there seems to have been some bias in the social class since over two-thirds were able to return to 'scholarly or professional' employment. In half the cases of coma this had exceeded 3 weeks. No direct relationship was found between duration of coma and the sequelae. These usually formed a complex syndrome in which psychological and neurological disabilities were closely associated. The pyramidal system was almost invariably affected and, if on both sides, much more markedly on one. On the less affected side there was often little more than an extensor plantar response and some awkwardness of movements of the upper limb, reminiscent of 'infantile' cerebral hemiplegias. Most of those with cerebellar involvement also had pyramidal signs, and there were three patients considered to have extrapyramidal disabilities combined with pyramidal deficits. Some impairment of sensory perception, usually involving an entire side, was found in just under a third of the patients, and in a small number this, or astereognosis with a tendency to ignore the hand, constituted the severest disability. In about a sixth of these cases there was severe slowness of speech due to pseudobulbar or cerebellar lesions, and, rarely, to palatal palsy.

The authors make the point that this slowness in speaking was often only one element in a general 'intellectual viscosity'. Intellectual function was impaired in just under half the patients. In only a few was this global and in most it could be more specifically defined. Amongst these a third of the patients were peculiarly 'slow in thought and the formulation of ideas', a quarter were defective in attention span and in most there was a disturbance of short-term memory. This slowness might not be apparent in the normal course of daily life but it constituted a profound disability in further training and later employment. Personality disorders characterised by disinhibition, which was often severely disabling, occurred frequently, as did aggression, apathy, depression and anxiety. The intensity of these personality changes declined with time and most became compatible with social life. The risk of suicide was high. The duration of coma in this series is carefully defined but the authors did not find any direct relationship between duration of coma and post-traumatic sequelae.

The period over which 42 patients from another rehabilitation unit were followed by Rodineau, Deseilligny, Bussel and Held (1970) varied between 6 weeks and 9 years, and again no clear reference is made to the effect which the time factor had on outcome. The authors did not consider that age or length of coma significantly affected 'functional prognosis' although, surprisingly, they qualify this by commenting that the results were often better when the coma was not prolonged. In patients who had severe spasticity and incoordination at the time of their admission to the unit the outlook for good functional recovery was poor, but there was good or satisfactory recovery of motor function in over two-thirds of their patients. In a sixth of the cases the persisting paresis and spasticity of an upper limb made it virtually useless. They observed that, on the whole, cerebellar syndromes tended to regress well. It is not clear what their selection criteria were, other than by admission to a unit for neural disabilities requiring rehabilitation.

In a study of the case records of 320 patients who regained consciousness and survived 1–10 years after closed head injury, Carlsson, Essen and Löfgren (1968) confine themselves to an examination of the predictive value of coma duration, age and sex. All the patients had been unconscious for longer than 12 hours, unconsciousness being defined as persisting until the patient responded verbally. Surgically treated cases were excluded. The authors' criterion of recovery was 'mental restitution', which they defined as the ability 'to work' or to 'look after themselves'. Recovery in these terms and the rate at which it occurred was found to be dependent upon age and duration of coma, and could be represented by a simple monoexponential curve. In all, 82 per cent were considered to have been 'restituted'. Restitution was independent of the duration of coma under the age of twenty years, and over that age 4 weeks of coma was the maximum consistent with restitution. For patients injured between the ages of twenty-one and fifty, all recovered in the way defined if coma had not lasted for longer than 24 hours. The 'probability of restitution' declined to 50 per cent if coma persisted for longer than a week and, in this age group, no patient unconscious for longer than 12 days 'was restituted'. In patients aged over fifty at the time of injury there was only a 50 per cent chance of restitution after coma lasting for more than $3\frac{1}{2}$ days.

Selection by Criterion of Age

The importance of age as a determinant of the long-term outlook for disabilities due to severe closed head injuries is stressed in most of the preceding reports concerning patients not specifically selected by age. There have been few studies confined to the late effects of accidental head injuries in children. In such papers the factor of age is examined in greater detail, but none of them attempts a specific comparison with adult series. Brink, Garrett, Hale, Woo-Sam and Nickel (1970) selected a series of children admitted to a rehabilitation unit who had been 'comatose' for more than a week, this term not being further defined. The 46 survivors were re-examined by the authors between 1 and 7 years after their injuries. The ages of the patients ranged from two to eighteen years, the median being eight years. The majority had initially been decerebrate or decorticate. Neurological disabilities were assessed in detail and it was found that spasticity and ataxia were the commonest major sequelae. Moderate to severe spasticity was nearly three times more common in patients who had been comatose for longer than a month. It was unilateral in about half the patients and bilateral in the remainder, although in the latter it was usually more severe on one side. Spasticity in all four limbs was much commoner where coma had exceeded a month. Ataxia was present in half the cases but was minimal in two-thirds of those affected. Only two patients were unable to walk because of the severity of their tetrapareses and ataxia, but a quarter of the total were limited to walking short distances. Nearly half the patients had persisting defects in articulation. Overall improvement was noted to continue for as long as 3 years after injury, but the maximum gains were achieved in the first year. The majority of these children became independent and able to care for themselves. On the other hand, scholastically the majority of patients remained 'impaired'. The younger the child at the time of injury the more pronounced were the intellectual deficits, but these did not seem to be more marked in the patients who had been unconscious longer than a month. Using standard Wechsler and Binet tests of intelligence it was shown, a year or more after injury, that two-thirds of these children were at or below the borderline retardation level. There was a substantial prevalence of behaviour disorder, of which the most common manifestations were hyperactivity, short attention span, temper tantrums and aggressive or destructive behaviour.

Flach and Malmros (1972) studied 131 children of whom none was older than thirteen at the time of injury. Eight to ten years later they were re-admitted to the neurosurgical unit in which they had initially been treated, for reassessment. Selection criteria are not clearly stated but the series appears to comprise all patients who were referred to the neurosurgical unit because they were considered to have suffered a head injury severe enough to warrant neurosurgical assessment at some stage after injury. The grading of severity takes into consideration two by no means closely related factors. The least severe are described as having suffered simple uncomplicated fractures or cerebral concussion, these amounting to a third of the patients. A further third had comminuted or depressed fractures with or without verified brain laceration or contusion, and these were subjected to an operation which is otherwise unspecified. The remainder were considered to have had severe diffuse cerebral oedema or 'brainstem' injury, or had suffered compression by extra or subdural haematoma. The authors' assessment of outcome was based on the extent to which the injured child had attained a social position corresponding to that of his siblings and parents.

In their first group of patients, described as having suffered relatively mild head injuries, one-fifth were classified as being maladjusted by this measure of social rehabilitation. A quarter of the children who were considered to exhibit unquestionable evidence of organic impairment were not, however, found to be maladjusted on tests of intellectual function. These were older at the time of injury than the other children and were thought to have compensated for their cognitive deficits at the expense of emotional development.

Their parents considered them to be immature. Loss of consciousness persisting for less than an hour, even in those who had sustained simple skull fractures, rarely left any serious disability. Coma lasting for 1–3 weeks was not incompatible with full mental and neurological recovery. Decerebrate attacks which continued for 3 weeks did not prevent a three-year-old boy from making a complete recovery. A highly characteristic feature of the socially maladjusted children was slowness of thought and movement. Measurable hypoplasia of one or two limbs was a sequel in a sixth of the cases. The most frequent residual defect was a decline in performance in standard tests of intellectual function. The authors did not encounter a single case of the personality disorder termed 'minimal brain damage', which is characterised by restlessness, impaired concentration, dependence and easy fatigue.

In a brief report Heiskanen and Kaste (1974) describe their assessment of 35 children, all under sixteen years of age, whom they personally examined between 4 and 10 years after severe head injuries. The majority were considered to have suffered cerebral contusion but a fifth of the cases were complicated by surface brain compression or intracerebral haematoma requiring surgery. All had been unconscious for longer than 24 hours, the median duration of coma being 9 days. Hemipareses were found to be still present in a third of cases, and the majority of these were also intellectually impaired as judged by school performance, five of them being classifiable as 'educationally subnormal'. There were two cases of homonymous field defects, presumably due to cerebral lesions, and there was evidence of optic nerve injury in three other patients. A residual third nerve palsy persisted in two children. On examining the relationship between persisting disability and duration of coma, the authors came to the conclusion that only exceptionally would a child make normal school progress after 2 weeks of unconsciousness. They comment that although the prognosis of severe head injury in children is certainly better than in adults it can hardly be described as 'good' in these cases.

Studies Attempting to Identify Prognostic Indices of Short-term Outcome in Severe Closed Head Injury

There are numerous reports of attempts to predict and assess the outcome of severe accidental head injury in terms of immediate mortality and of the recovery taking place within a year or two of the injury. An exceptionally thorough analysis of the manner in which the type of traumatic coma exceeding 24 hours is related to outcome in the short-term is reported by Pazzaglia, Frank, Frank and Gaist (1975). Coma was judged to persist until there was some verbal response. Every patient was subjected to angiography. Although in no sense an assessment of long-term prognosis – so far as can be judged from the information provided – the authors' belief that it is possible to predict final outcome at an early stage after head injury warrants attention here. Of the 142 survivors examined over 2 years after injury, two-thirds were able to lead the same kind of social life they had led prior to injury, and in less than a quarter was the patient unable to support himself or to take care of his own daily needs. In substantially more than half the cases there were no residual sequelae. In a little less than a third there were mild sequelae which are referred to only in general terms as a 'partial deficit' of a cranial nerve, some degree of defective memory, 'mental inefficiency', or infrequent epileptic attacks. Typically these did not prevent the patient from leading the same kind of social life he had led prior to injury. Even in the fifth who were described as having marked sequelae, that is, a severe amnesic syndrome or language disturbance, dementia, a complete cranial nerve palsy, a motor deficit of one or more limbs, or epilepsy with frequent seizures, the disabilities were not invariably incompatible with normal social rehabilitation.

Using a classification of grades of coma based on Plum and Posner (1972), which, it should be noted here, is not always interpreted in the same way by all the authors who use it, they find that amongst those patients who reach a level of 'mesencephalic coma' only one-tenth recover completely. More 'caudal' grades of coma were invariably fatal in their patients, recovery mostly only being complete in the more 'rostral' types of coma. The authors do not further examine the significance of duration of coma. In the least severe grades of coma increasing age lessened the chance of complete recovery, and in mesencephalic coma only those under the age of forty years had any chance of recovering fully. Surgically treatable cerebral lacerations and brain compression by surface collections of blood carried a less favourable prognosis than uncomplicated injuries, with the single exception of chronic subdural haematomata.

In contrast Gutterman and Shenkin (1970) fail to define in any detail their concept of the traumatic decerebration suffered by the 52 consecutive patients they studied. The outcome was assessed between 3 months and 5 years after the injury in 29 survivors by examining the neurosurgical notes made during the period that the patients were being routinely followed up after the injury. In half the cases this had been complicated by intracranial haematomata. The duration of decerebration in those who were not treated surgically varied between 4 days and 4 months, and those with only slight or no residual deficit had been decerebrate for less than 3 weeks on average. However, 7 weeks of 'decerebration', not otherwise qualified, was compatible with slight residual deficits. Over half of these patients were children between the ages of five and fifteen. Severe neurological disability tended to be associated with longer decerebration, 6 weeks on average, but only 4 days of decerebration could be followed by moderately severe neurological disabilities. The short-lived decerebration associated with surgically treatable surface brain compression was not usually followed by severe neural lesions.

In a study aimed principally at distinguishing the predictive value of various neural syndromes of decerebration in terms of death or survival, Pagni (1973) comments in passing, and without citing figures, on the long-term prospects for mental and physical recovery. The 471 patients who became decerebrate after accidental head injury represented 43 per cent of all head injuries admitted over less than 10 years to a neurosurgical unit. Complete recovery without sequelae was never observed if decerebration of any kind had persisted for longer than a fortnight. Complete recovery had been observed in short-lasting 'mesencephalic' decerebration in which cranial nerve brainstem reflexes were preserved, but only if the injury was not complicated by intracranial space occupying lesions. In all cases of 'mesencephalo-pontine' decerebration in which cranial nerve brainstem reflexes were abnormal or depressed but not lost, there were mental or physical sequelae, that is with the exception of some surgically treated cases. The number of patients without sequelae after traumatic decerebration declined with increasing age.

In an examination of the prognostic significance, in the short term, of the patient's neurological status as recorded at the first examination on admission to hospital, Overgaard, Hvid-Hansen, Land, Pedersen, Christensen, Haase, Hein and Tweed (1973) studied a consecutive series of 138 survivors of 'blunt' head injury. They assessed separately the level of arousal in response to stimulation and the characteristics of the motor response provoked, and then compared these with the outcome. A distinction was made between a 'coordinated' and a decerebrate response. The latter was further subdivided into 'typical rigidity', in which there was pronation of the arms together with extension of all four limbs, and 'atypical rigidity', which included all other 'abnormal extensor and rotary motor responses'. These latter might be elicited in the limbs on only one side and be associated with a 'coordinated' response in one or more of the other extremities.

The authors identified these motor responses to stimulation as the most important single factor associated with outcome in injury sustained before the age of thirty years. In the absence of decerebration, either 'typical' or 'atypical', over two-thirds of the patients recovered fully or with only minor 'deficits'. Decerebration over the age of thirty was never associated with this grade of recovery. Post-traumatic hypertension of over 160 mm Hg in both younger and older age groups was associated with a greater incidence of 'severe deficits', as were complicated injuries requiring neurosurgical treat-ment. The upper age limits for good recovery after decerebration were found to be ten years when this was 'typical' and twenty years when it was 'atypical' rigidity. Since the early neurological state correlated so well with outcome, and the authors found that this state changed little in most patients who survived the first week, it was felt that the maximum brain damage occurred within minutes or hours after severe head injury. The authors do not attempt to make any assessment of the effect which either the duration of coma or these levels of motor responsiveness had on outcome.

In preliminary reports of a continuing prospective study of factors predict-ing outcome in the short-term and determining management in the acute post-traumatic period, Jennett and his many colleagues have similarly shown the close relationship between, and predictive value of, 'motor responsiveness, verbal performance and eye opening' (Teasdale and Jennett, 1974; Jennett, Teasdale and Knill-Jones, 1975; Jennett, Teasdale, Galbraith, Pickard, Grant, Braakman, Avezaat, Maas, Minderhoud, Vecht, Heiden, Small, Caton, and Kurze, 1977). Using a system of summed scores for each of these and other variables at successive stages after injury, and examining the worst and the best 'levels of coma' assessed in this manner, the authors show that the 'best' level of motor responsiveness is a 'potent predictor in the first week'.

In seeking a more objective and less clinically dependent method of distinguishing, at an early stage after injury, between patients who will make an acceptable recovery and those who will survive only as 'vegetative wrecks', Vapalahti and Troupp (1971) used measurements of intracranial pressure and of blood gas tensions in a prospective study of 50 patients. In showing that these were valuable indices of prognosis for death or survival the authors nevertheless note that in patients over the age of twenty years it is the clinically observable constellation of decerebration, periodic respiration and hyperthermia together with laboratory evidence of respiratory alkalosis, which most accurately predicts that survival will be only in a vegetative state.

As Brierley and Excell (1966) and Brierley (1971) have shown, the pathological end-results of severe acute hypoxia are the same as those which follow cardiac arrest. Essentially, both culminate in cerebral perfusion failure causing damage which is maximal in the watershed territory between the areas of supply of the major cerebral vessels, and also in areas supplied by individual arteries, especially if these are abnormal in any way. This same pattern of pathological brain damage has been shown by Graham and Adams (1971) to be an unexpectedly frequent finding in the brains of patients who die as a result of severe closed head injury. As will be discussed later, there is also good clinical evidence to suggest that cerebral perfusion failure is an important contributory factor in brain damage amongst those who survive. In passing, therefore, it would seem pertinent to note here the observations made by Willoughby and Leach (1974) on the close association between the neurological state of the patient 1 hour after cardiac arrest and the short-term outcome. In a study of 48 patients followed up between 2 weeks and 18 months after cardiac arrest, these authors showed that total unresponsiveness to stimulation or decerebrate posturing at 1 hour or more after injury, is followed by death or survival with varying degrees of neurological disability. In that the latter ranged from acute akinesia to a degree of memory impairment which did not prevent employment under supervision, this method of assessment cannot be held to be highly discriminatory in respect of the nature and degree of disability. It would seem likely that a larger series of patients and further subdivision of the levels of neural responsiveness and their duration, as has been attempted after head injury, might enable a more accurate prediction to be made of possible disability in survivors. Again, as in head injury, the duration of coma has been found to have predictive value after cardiac arrest, Bokonjic and Buchthal (1961) having shown that 'post-anoxic' coma lasting less than 2 days was followed by complete recovery.

In the majority of the above reports which attempt to relate severity of injury to outcome the two principal defects are the failure, first, to identify the natural history of each component of the mental and neurophysical disabilities following severe closed head injury, and second, to suggest characteristics of the early post-traumatic state which would help in estimating the likely prognosis for each of these in the individual case.

In addition to the studies reviewed above there are numerous reports of the long-term outcome after severe closed head injury in which, despite much valuable information and comment on the subject, the limitations of design or method of investigation are such that they do not add materially to the facts derived from the reports already summarised. Included amongst these are the studies reported by Rowbotham (1949), Akerlund (1959) and Heiskanen and Sipponen (1970). In these the majority of patients were followed up only by postal questionnaire, a method which is not likely to produce reliable data on the subject of domestic, social and occupational rehabilitation. Amongst many others, the otherwise valuable contributions of London (1967) and Lewin (1965, 1966, 1968a,b, 1970), which deal with the problem of long-term outcome only in passing within the general context of disability due to head injury, do not add to the reports already cited which are specifically concerned with long-term prognosis. These and other studies are referred to again in the text when they are relevant to discussion of the results.

3 Method of Patient Selection and Design of the Investigation

Method of Patient Selection

The principal purpose of this study was to assess the long-term effect of a single head injury in a series of patients, unselected except by clearly defined criteria of severity. It was also intended that every patient included in the study should be traced and all the survivors examined. Similarly, the cause of death was to be established in every case dying since the injury so that any effect the head injury had on life expectancy could be determined. In general terms, therefore, this was designed as an epidemiological study of an unselected sample of patients with the severest injuries from a population of patients who had sustained head injury considered serious enough to warrant their admission to hospital. In this way it was hoped to avoid the type of selection bias which limits the value of many previously reported studies, prevents comparisons between one study and another, and makes it difficult to formulate general statements about the ultimate outcome for specific neural disabilities which follow severe non-missile brain injury.

The selection requirements were met by the provision of a population totalling 7000 patients who had been admitted consecutively between 1948 and 1961 to the Accident and Neurosurgical Services of the Radcliffe Infirmary, Oxford. In each case the identifying data, a note of the complications, treatment, progress in convalescence and short-term outcome, together with an assessment of the duration of the post-traumatic amnesia, were available on punchcards. These were the personal collection of Mr Walpole Lewin, reflecting his continuing interest in the management of head injuries over these years.

From among these consecutive 7000 cases, every patient injured between five and eighty-five years of age and recorded as having a post-traumatic amnesia lasting a week or longer was selected for study. In addition an examination was made of all punchcards on which the duration of the post-traumatic amnesia had not been recorded. In the majority of these cases the patient had failed to recover sufficiently from his head injury for the length of post-traumatic amnesia to be established, or the severity of the head injury had been such that the patient had been transferred to another hospital whilst still amnesic or unconscious, so that information about subsequent examinations had not been indexed. With the few exceptions of these patients transferred to other hospitals, an assessment of the length of post-traumatic amnesia was found to have been made and recorded in the hospital notes at the time of later examinations.

Since any patient who had remained unconscious for longer than a week would have had amnesia for this length of time, these were also selected for inclusion in the study. Those who recalled a lucid interval were excluded. In the most severely injured and demented no assessment of post-traumatic amnesia had been possible, but since this had evidently extended for longer than a week these cases were also included in the study. All patients who developed intracranial infection, or who had sustained spinal cord or brachial plexus lesions in addition to head injury, were excluded. A small number of American ex-servicemen were also excluded because costs would have prevented any contact other than by the totally inadequate method of follow-up assessment by postal questionnaires. A number of Polish and Yugoslavian nationals were excluded after the first three patients had been re-examined. It became clear that no useful purpose was likely to be served by attempting to assess the social rehabilitation of a group of patients who remained socially and culturally isolated from their adopted community, and still unable to speak its language after 25 years' residence.

In the period under review, admission to the Accident Service of the Radcliffe Infirmary was arranged after head injury if there was evidence of cerebral concussion, judged by a period of post-traumatic amnesia, or if there was a skull fracture or severe scalp laceration. The majority of cases, that is 80 per cent, were admitted direct from the scene of the accident within an hour, or from the casualty departments of other hospitals within a few hours of injury, because this was the only hospital in the area admitting accidents. The remaining 20 per cent were transferred from other hospitals outside the immediate area when neurosurgical treatment was evidently necessary or the condition of the patient was such as to raise the possibility that it might be needed. The population of head injured patients from which the present series is drawn is therefore typical of the general population of patients suffering accidental head injuries in peacetime and handled by an accident service providing specialist neurosurgical cover. Generalisations based on this assumption will be made later.

The patients were in the care of an orthopaedic surgeon and a neurosurgeon, and were supervised from the outset by a neurosurgical team. The information recorded was therefore uniform and the evaluation and descriptions of the patients' neurological states were detailed and reliable.

A total of 479 patients was selected for study. Throughout the following text these will be referred to as the *consecutive series* of patients. To this consecutive series were added 69 patients who had survived an accidental head injury which had caused unconsciousness lasting a month or longer. These were the personal series of Mr Walpole Lewin, treated between 1948 and 1970 in his practice as neurosurgeon to the British Army and at the Addenbrooke's Hospital, Cambridge. In this study the patient was assumed to be unconscious until he showed some comprehension of the spoken word. The majority of these patients were unresponsive, apart from various forms of decerebrate and other reflex posturing, for at least a month. The details of the level of coma and type of neural response to stimulation will be given later.

The 40 survivors examined, combined with the 24 from the consecutive series who survived in coma a month and were followed up, are the *selected series*.

In tracing these patients, the consecutive series between 10 and 24 years, and the selected series between 3 and 25 years after their injuries, it was found that the original recorded addresses served only as a general guide to the area in which enquiry should be made. Assistance was sought from various registers, including those of the National Health and Social Security Services, whose officials undertook to forward letters to patients whom they were able to trace. Examination of the archives of the General Register Office and local street and telephone directories provided helpful information. A substantial proportion of the patients were traced only after diligent and time-consuming house-to-house enquiries made by social workers and other helpers. A total of 538 patients was traced in this way. Three were lost to the survey because the original case records could not be found. One was lost to the survey because, although traced, he refused to be examined. Of the remaining seven who could not be traced, six were from the consecutive and one from the selected series.

Table 3.1   The patients included in the study

TOTAL SERIES	
Radcliffe unselected consecutive (PTA 1 week or more) and Army and Addenbrooke's selected (coma 1 month or more)	548
Lost	11
Traced	537
Dead	206
Total examined	331
Consecutive series	479
Lost	10
Traced	469
Dead Uncomplicated	98
Complicated	80
Examined Uncomplicated	214
Complicated	77
Total examined	291
Selected series (coma 1 month or more)	69
Army and Addenbrooke's	
Lost	1
Dead Uncomplicated	19
Complicated	9
Examined Uncomplicated	27
Complicated	13
Total examined	40
Radcliffe consecutive	
Examined	24
Combined selected total examined	64

It was found that 206 were no longer alive. The cause of death in each case was established from information made available by the General Register Office, general practitioners, hospital records or relatives.

In table 3.1 these details of the patients selected for inclusion in the study are summarised.

The surviving 331 patients were invited by letter to attend for interview and re-examination at the London Hospital, Addenbrooke's Hospital, Cambridge or the Radcliffe Infirmary, Oxford, whichever was the more convenient. Each patient was asked to bring a close relative to provide an independent account. An independent account was made available in this way for 82 per cent of cases in the consecutive series and for 93 per cent of cases in the selected series. This often came from two sources, both spouse and parent, when it was apparent that one or the other was able to give only a part of the story. There were 42 patients who declined or failed to attend and had to be visited in their homes. Only one refused to be examined when called upon. He is included among the 11 lost to the survey. With a single exception all of the 291 survivors of the consecutive series were examined personally by the author, as were all except five of the 40 survivors in the selected series. These five patients were still under regular review by Mr Walpole Lewin, and his case notes were used for their follow-up assessments.

Design of the Investigation

Each patient interviewed by the author was asked the same set of questions, the answers to which were entered on standard forms designed for the study. His spontaneous description of his residual disabilities was complemented by a series of questions designed to elicit information about epileptic phenomena, vestibular disturbances and headache, and about sexual and bladder function. He was asked his view of his tolerance to alcohol. His own assessment of his memory both for day-to-day and past events was sought in detail; and he was asked to comment on the ease or difficulty with which, in his opinion, he expressed himself verbally or comprehended what was said to him both in the first few months after the accident and subsequently. Symptoms of disturbed right hemisphere function were sought by asking the patient if he had been aware of any difficulty in finding his way about familiar or unfamiliar places or in recognising faces since the injury. Finally each was asked to describe with what ease or difficulty he had adjusted to study or to learning the requirements of new jobs since his injury.

The period he believed he had been away from work after his injury was checked where possible from other sources. The question of litigation and compensation and the sums of money involved were noted. A detailed past medical and family history was taken, the latter including the social class of his parents and siblings, and the incidence of psychiatric, epileptic and neurological disorders amongst them. Each was questioned about his marriage, the ages, health and occupation of his children, and about domestic harmony or otherwise.

An assessment of personality change after the injury was then made on the basis of the answers given by the patient to a series of questions concerning levels of social anxiety and phobic symptoms, irritability and aggressiveness, mood swings, paranoid ideas of reference or feelings of suspicion, and sociability or solitariness before and after the injury. Comparison was then made with the description of personality change given by spouse or parent. The patient was asked to recall in detail the various jobs he had held before and after his accident, the length of time he had spent in each, and his reasons for leaving. Information was also recorded concerning schooling and scholastic achievement, and where applicable about service and rank in the armed forces. Details of university education and academic distinctions were noted.

The patient was then submitted to a neurological examination, the observations again being recorded on a standard form covering verbal functions, articulation, cranial nerve functions, mental state including a comment on rapport, mood and paranoid ideation or attitudes observed at interview. Motor and sensory function, coordination and equilibrium were then assessed in the usual way, and this was followed by a brief systemic examination. At each stage in this clinical assessment of neural function the patient was asked his view of his disabilities as each system was being examined. During this examination of the patient, relatives, if available, were interviewed independently by a psychiatric social worker, Mrs Dorothy Weir, about the patient, using a questionnaire designed for the study. Details of the accident, if known to them, were noted together with information about any compensation paid and after what delay. The previous health of the patient, his occupational and social status, including details of his schooling, interests and hobbies, were recorded. The relatives' recollection of the disabilities present at the time of discharge from hospital in the spheres of coordination, balance, vision, speech, memory and intellectual impairment were then sought. The relative was asked if there had been or still were complaints of headache, episodes of altered consciousness, changes in personality or in domestic and social behaviour or interests, and to comment on any alterations in sexual performance. Each was encouraged to recall the length of time it had taken for the disabilities most evident to them to improve or resolve, and how long that improvement had continued. Observations they had made of either mental or physical deterioration after initial improvement were noted. Finally, relatives were asked to comment in general on explanations given to them by medical and nursing staff to help them cope with difficult behaviour and physical disability, and to air their views on the rehabilitation facilities offered.

An assessment was made of the quality and reliability of the information provided in this way. Points of interest arising out of these interviews were discussed with the author, who then interviewed relatives further on specific points as seemed necessary.

Over three-quarters of the patients were then submitted to a series of tests of intellectual function and memory by a clinical psychologist, Dr Eileen Smith. These tests were selected from among those found by Newcombe (1969) to be sensitive to impaired cognitive functions in a series of patients brain-damaged by penetrating missile wounds. They were designed to provide an overall assessment of intelligence and then specifically to examine those functions which are held to be lateralised to left and right cerebral hemispheres.

An estimate of the Intelligence Quotient was made using Raven's Progressive Matrices and the synonym selection test of the Mill Hill vocabulary (Raven, 1958).

Four tests were used to assess verbal and verbal memory functions. The first of these was an object naming test described by Oldfield and Wingfield (1965). This involves the independent presentation of 36 outline drawings of objects, the names of which fall into word frequency ranges derived from the Thorndyke–Lorge count (Thorndyke and Lorge, 1944). Two measures were taken: the number of items correctly named, converted to percentages, and the time taken in milliseconds for each item to be named, designated the latency. Speed was emphasised and inability to produce the name within 4 seconds scored as failure. In the second test two short stories from the Wechsler memory scale (Wechsler, 1945) were read to the patient, who had to recall as much of each as possible after the presentation of each passage. This is referred to as immediate verbal recall. One hour later, and without warning, the patient again had to recall the story, and this constituted the delayed verbal recall. In both cases the score was the average number of items recalled. In the third test a series of numbers was presented verbally and the patient required to repeat them in the order in which they were given; after successful repetition a further digit was added until the patient had reached the limit of his ability to register and recall. Finally, a paired association learning test was taken from the Wechsler memory scale. Each patient had ten pairs of words with increasingly less obvious associations read to him, and was asked to memorise and recall them both immediately and after a delay.

Three tests of visuospatial function were used. These included the Block Design of the Wechsler Adult Intelligence Scale (Wechsler, 1944), which was administered and scored in the usual manner; the Wechsler designs, again taken from the Wechsler memory scale and given as described in the manual, measuring delayed and immediate recall; and finally a paper and pencil maze test described by Elithorne, Kerr and Jones (1963) in which the patient has to trace a pathway through a series of black dots placed on the vertices of criss-crossing diagonal lines. In the right-hand corner of each maze there is a number which informs the patient of the maximum number of dots he must incorporate for successful completion of the test. After three demonstrations the patient was allowed 2 minutes to complete each maze test. Three consecutive failures concluded the test. Scoring was by division of the number of mazes correctly done by the number attempted, and a total testing time of 12 minutes was allowed.

These, rather than more individually designed tests, were chosen so that comparisons could be made with patients tested similarly in previously reported assessments of cognitive deficits after head injury. They were limited in number in order that no more than $1\frac{1}{2}$ hours would be required to test a patient who, it was felt, might well become fatigued if subjected to longer examination at a single sitting.

4 The Patients and their Injuries

The following chapters provide first a general description of the two series of patients, consecutive and selected, included in the study, and then a detailed examination of the various disabilities, grouped separately in order to reveal how each contributes to the persisting overall incapacity. In each case the findings are considered in the light of other published clinical studies, and in relation to current concepts of the mechanics and pathology of cerebral trauma.

To preserve the epidemiological aspects of this study so that later estimates can be made of the number of patients with similar long persisting disabilities in the community, the two series of patients are initially considered separately. In the combined total of 548 patients, the 11 untraced patients (10 from the consecutive series and one from the selected series) are excluded from further consideration.

Table 3.1 shows that there was a total of 469 patients who had been admitted consecutively to one accident service after a head injury which had caused a post-traumatic amnesia or unconsciousness lasting for longer than a week. Of these, 291 were alive at the time of the study and, with a single exception, were examined personally by the author. Their ages at the time of injury and re-examination, and the period between are set out in table 4.1 and shown diagrammatically in figures 4.1 and 4.3. The details of the 178 dead are considered later in chapter 12.

Of the 69 patients selected from various sources whose injuries had caused unconsciousness persisting for longer than a month, 40 were alive at the time of the study and were re-examined. The details of the 28 dead are considered in the later chapter dealing with life expectancy and causes of death. The ages at the time of injury of the 40 survivors examined, together with the 24 patients from the consecutive series who survived similar prolonged unconsciousness, are set out in table 4.2. The age distribution at the time of injury and review, and the time between in this combined series of 64 patients is illustrated in figures 4.2 and 4.3.

Various measures of the severity of the head injury sustained by the 291 patients in the consecutive series re-examined 10−24 years after their injuries, and the proportion of patients involved in each case, are illustrated in table 4.3 and figure 4.4. The same information for the selected series of patients is set out in table 4.4 and figure 4.5.

A *complicated* injury was defined as one in which surgical treatment had been required for traumatic brain penetration, or in which surgical treatment had involved removal of brain substance. It also included those cases treated surgically in which there had been surface brain compression by subdural haematomata or hygromata and extradural haematomata. The definition

Table 4.1   Ages at injury and re-examination and time elapsed between in consecutive series survivors (total 291 patients)

| | Age (years) | | | | | |
	5–15	16–25	26–35	36–45	46–55	56+
Uncomplicated						
At injury	39	81	32	30	21	11
At follow up	0	26	62	53	26	47
Complicated						
At injury	9	20	20	10	15	3
At follow up	0	5	13	23	11	25
Uncomplicated and complicated at injury						
Number of patients	48	101	52	40	36	14
Percentage	17%	35%	18%	14%	12%	5%
Uncomplicated and complicated at follow up						
Number of patients	0	31	75	76	37	72
Percentage	0	11%	26%	26%	13%	25%
Years between injury and follow-up examination						
10–15 years						
Number of patients	80		56		32	
Percentage	28%		19%		11%	
16–24 years						
Number of patients	69		36		18	
Percentage	24%		12%		6%	

excludes those cases in which exploratory burr holes were made but there was no confirmation of surface brain compression, cases in which surgical treatment had been required for depressed fractures where the dura remained intact, and also patients who had surgical penetration of the brain solely by needle for assessment or ventriculography. The incidence of these complications is set out in table 4.5.

Unconsciousness was defined as persisting until the patient showed some comprehension of the spoken word by obeying a verbal request.

A response to stimulation in the unconscious patient which consisted of tonic extension of one or both legs, together with tonic extension or flexion of one or both arms, was considered *decerebrate* and to have persisted until semipurposive or purposive movements were recorded.

The length of the *post-traumatic amnesia* had been assessed and recorded in the hospital notes by various members of the neurosurgical teams involved in the care of the patient at varying intervals after the injury, and was uniformly defined after Russell (1932). It was assumed to persist until there was restoration of full orientation and normal registration and recall of day-to-day

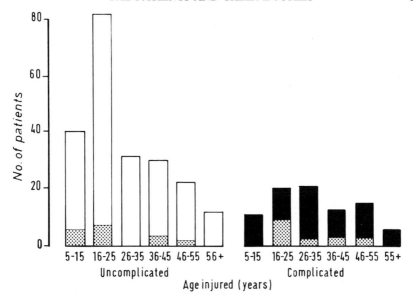

Figure 4.1   The ages at injury of the 291 surviving patients in the consecutive series who were unconscious or amnesic for a week or more. Note that the stippled areas refer to the 24 patients within this group who were unconscious for more than a month.

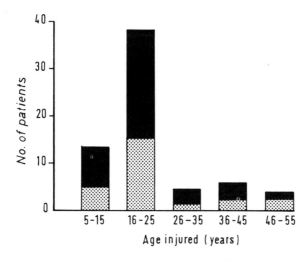

Figure 4.2   The ages at injury of the 64 surviving patients in the selected series who were unconscious for a month or more. Note that the stippled areas refer to the 22 complicated cases within this group.

Table 4.2   Ages at injury and re-examination and time elapsed between in selected
series survivors (total 64 patients)

| | Age (years) | | | | | |
	5–15	16–25	26–35	36–45	46–55	56+
At injury						
Number of patients	13	38	4	5	4	0
Percentage	20%	60%	6%	8%	6%	
At follow up						
Number of patients	4	14	25	12	6	3
Percentage	6%	22%	39%	19%	9%	5%
Years between injury and						
follow up examination						
3–5 years						
Number of patients		15			2	
Percentage		23%			3%	
6–10 years						
Number of patients		16			4	
Percentage		25%			6%	
11+ years						
Number of patients		24			3	
Percentage		38%			5%	

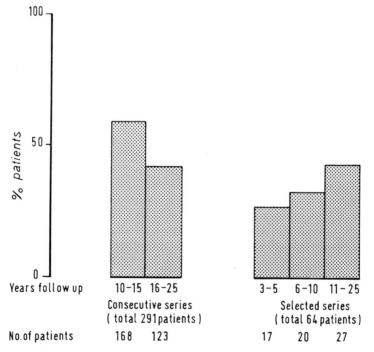

Figure 4.3   The time (in years) between injury and follow-up examination for the 331
surviving patients from the consecutive and selected series.

Table 4.3 Measures of severity of injury of survivors of consecutive series of 291 patients re-examined between 10 and 24 years after injury

	Age injured (years)						Totals
	5–15	16–25	26–35	36–45	46–55	56+	
Totals	48	101	52	40	36	14	291
Uncomplicated	39	81	32	30	21	11	214
Complicated	9	20	20	10	15	3	77
Duration PTA							
1 week +							
Number of patients	11	32	16	9	11	3	82
Percentage	23%	32%	31%	23%	31%		
2–3 weeks +							
Number of patients	23	35	22	14	12	3	110
Percentage	48%	35%	44%	34%	33%	21%	38%
4 weeks +							
Number of patients	14	34	14	17	13	8	99
Percentage	29%	33%	25%	43%	36%	58%	34%
Duration coma							
Up to 1 week							
Number of patients	15	49	30	18	24	7	143
Percentage	31%	49%	58%	45%	67%	50%	48%
1+ up to 4 weeks							
Number of patients	29	39	21	20	8	7	124
Percentage	60%	38%	40%	50%	22%	50%	40%
1 month +							
Number of patients	4	13	1	2	4	0	24
Percentage	9%	13%	2%	5%	11%		12%
Duration decerebration (total)							63
1 day or less							
Number of patients	0	7	6	4	0	0	17
Percentage							6%
2 days to less than 1 week							
Number of patients	11	11	3	2	3	0	30
Percentage							10%
1 week or more							
Number of patients	6	6	1	3	0	0	16
Percentage							6%

Table continued overleaf

Table 4.3—*continued*

	Age injured (years)						Totals
	5–15	16–25	26–35	36–45	46–55	56+	
Severe neurophysical disability in convalescence							
Number of patients unable to walk at 6 weeks unassisted due to neural lesions	9	17	6	7	10		49 (17%)
Number of patients unable to walk at 2 months unassisted due to neural lesions	6	13	5	6	7		37 (13%)

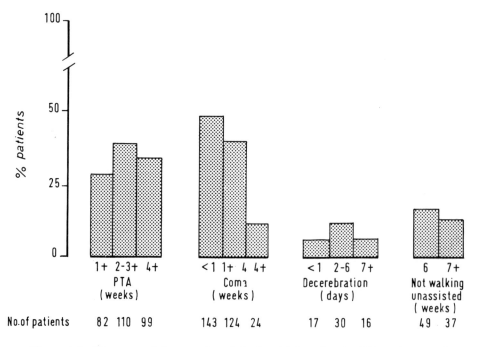

Figure 4.4 Measures of the severity of the head injury for the 291 patients in the consecutive series.

Table 4.4   Measures of severity of injury in survivors of selected series of 64 patients re-examined between 3 and 25 years after injury

	Age injured (years)				Totals	%
	5–15	16–35	36–45	46+		
Duration PTA						
Up to 12 weeks						
Number of patients	8	15	1	1	25	39%
13–24 weeks						
Number of patients	1	11	1	1	14	22%
25 weeks + or permanent						
Number of patients	4	16	3	2	25	39%
Duration coma						
4–6 weeks						
Number of patients	11	19	2	2	34	53%
6 weeks+						
Number of patients	2	23	3	2	30	47%
Duration decerebration						
Up to 2 weeks						
Number of patients	10	28	2	2	42	65%
2 weeks+						
Number of patients	2	11	2	0	15	23%
Severe neurological disability in convalescence						
Number of patients unable to walk unassisted due to neural lesions until 3–6 months	3	12	1	0	16	25%
Number of patients unable to walk unassisted due to neural lesions until 6 months or permanently	10	30	4	4	48	75%

Table 4.5   Type of complication of head injury in survivors of both series of patients

	Surface compression (subdural* or extradural haematoma or hygroma)	Brain penetration (surgical or traumatic and surface compression)	Traumatic brain penetration alone	Vascular†
Consecutive series	39 (16)Ex	13 (2)Ex	21	4
Selected series	9 (3)Ex	1 (1)Ex	4	0

* *Subdurals* all evacuated within first week except eight, of which four were evacuated within 10 days.
( ) Ex, Extradural haematoma.
† Occlusion internal carotid or branch, or major sinus thrombosis.

events. The management of these patients has been described by Lewin (1966). A total of 34 patients in the consecutive series was treated with a tracheostomy, as were 37 in the selected series. Hypothermia or cooling were employed as seemed indicated.

Table 4.6   Incidence of fractures of the skull in both series of patients

| | Age at injury (years) | | | | |
	5–15	16–35	36–45	46+	Totals
Consecutive series					
Total number of patients	48	153	40	50	291
Number of patients with					
skull fractures	32	94	29	37	192
Percentage					65%
Selected series					
Total number of patients	13	42	5	4	64
Number of patients with					
skull fractures	7	25	1	2	35
Percentage					55%

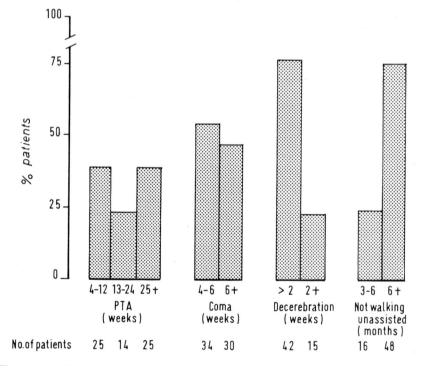

Figure 4.5   Measures of the severity of the head injury for the 64 patients in the selected series.

The type of accident and the incidence of skull fractures are recorded for these two series of patients in tables 4.6 and 4.7. There were 215 males in the consecutive and 40 in the selected series.

Table 4.7   Type of accident in both series of patients

	Consecutive series (291 patients)		Selected series (64 patients)	
	Totals	%	Totals	%
Motorcycle rider or pillion	111	38%	17	27%
Bicycle rider	65	22%	7	11%
Vehicle driver or passenger	36	12%	13	20%
Pedestrian versus vehicle	40	14%	18	28%
Fall	20	7%	6	10%
Horse	10	3%	2	3%
Other	9	3%	1	2%

Discussion

It is apparent that the severity of the injury sustained by the patients in this study is, in general, substantially greater for a larger proportion than in the previously reported studies of long-term prognosis reviewed earlier.

It is also clear that, although the definition of post-traumatic amnesia used here is that universally applied, definitions of *coma, decerebration* and *complication* differ from those used by a number of other authors; indeed there are also variations in definitions of these terms in the reports of many of the authors already cited. In their review of the short-term outcome of severe head injury Carlsson, Essen and Löfgren (1968) considered that the patient remained unconscious 'until he responded verbally, however inadequately, to the spoken word'. This, as in the definition used in the present study, leaves unresolved the problem of failure to comprehend or speak because of focal damage in the dominant hemisphere. Subdivision of the type of verbal response to stimulation, as suggested by Teasdale and Jennett (1974), goes no further in determining the contribution made by impairment of verbal functions to 'unconsciousness' defined in this way, though it may enable more accurate comparisons to be made between one study and another.

Similarly there are varying definitions to be found for the concept of decerebrate responses to stimulation in the unconscious patient. In the present study it could not be consistently relied upon that for each patient noted in the clinical records as responding with decerebrate posturing there would be a full description of its type, although this was so in the majority of cases. Thus it seemed wisest to classify as decerebrate all cases referred to in more or less detail as decerebrate and to assume that this state persisted until specific mention was made of semipurposive or purposive movements developing in a limb. It is probable that much has been lost in this way that would have been of value had it been possible to discriminate between various types of decerebration, as did Overgaard, Christensen, Hvid-Hansen, Haase, Land, Hein, Pedersen and Tweed (1973) in their short-term retrospective study of the outcome of severe head injury. These authors distinguished between classical decerebrate extension of all four limbs and the partial variants of the syndrome in which there was spontaneous or evoked flexion or semipurposive movements of one or more limbs. In the coma scale which they recommend, Teasdale and Jennett (1974) make a similar plea for a clearly defined record of motor responsiveness to stimulation which will be an indication of 'the functional state of the brain as a whole'. They record 'the best or highest response from any limb' in their graded scale of motor responsiveness to stimulation. A less precise reference to 'extension rigidity' is made by Vapalahti and Troupp (1971), who rely, however, on intracranial pressure studies and gas tensions in addition to clinical criteria for their prognostic indices of short-term outcome in patients with severe brain injuries.

It has to be accepted that in any retrospective study where clinical descriptions of neural signs are sought it is unlikely that a clear account will be found of all that is required many years later. In fact it is more than likely that any hospital records used in attempts to predict long-term outcome, even those from centres with a special interest and expertise in the neurological management of head injury, will suffer from the same deficiencies. It is possible, therefore, that despite these shortcomings predictive data which do not depend upon too subtle a degree of discrimination might have a wider application in the overall problem of assessing prognosis after head injury in the community.

5 Patterns of Residual Central Neural Lesions and Associated Disabilities

In this chapter only those neural lesions causing physical disabilities which are the result of damage to brain, cerebellum and brainstem are considered. The selection criteria excluded patients whose head injuries had been complicated by spinal cord and brachial plexus injury. At the time of re-examination none had evidence of such an injury that had been overlooked. The term 'central neural' is obviously a personal one, but by using it the intention is to exclude at this stage disabilities due to cranial and other peripheral nerve lesions, and also traumatic personality change and impaired intellectual function. These are better considered separately (chapters 7 and 9).

It was possible to recognise four principal patterns or constellations of signs of neural damage in these two series of patients. Figure 5.1 represents typical

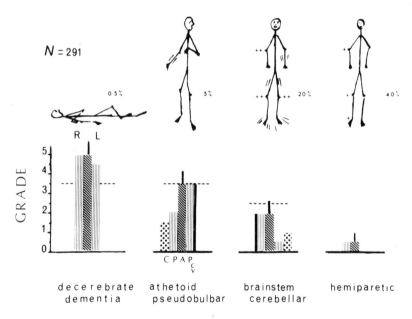

Figure 5.1   Central neural disability profiles.

cases of each in the form of histograms, each bar indicating the evidence of disturbed function found in a neural system, graded in terms of the degree of disability it caused as defined in table 5.1. The central bar in the histogram of each pattern or syndrome scores axial akinesia, disequilibrium, and, in the case of the less severely injured, dysarthria. On either side of the central bar

Table 5.1   Assessment of central neural disability

Grade	Score	Neural responsiveness in acute period and/or physical disability thereafter
Decerebrate dementia	5	
Purposive or semi-purposive response to stimulation	4.5	
Total dependence	4	Bed- or chairbound
	3.5	Ambulant only with the assistance of another person
Profound disability	3	Dense hemiparesis, akinesia, ataxia or disequilibrium but mobile without assistance. All *precluding* normal domestic, social *or* occupational life
Severe disability	2.5	As above. All *limiting substantially* normal domestic, social *or* occupational life
Moderate disability	2	Hemiparesis, spasticity, incoord-ination, dysarthria or imbalance. All causing *difficulties* with mobility or other physical activities in household, or social life, or job
Slight disability	1.5	As above, but *inconvenient* only
Minimal disability	1	Awareness of some slight defect of coordination, power, sensibility, articulation or balance of *little significance* in the home, socially or at work
Negligible disability	0.5	Abnormal physical signs only
No disability	0	

the disturbance of pyramidal function is represented by a bar for left and right limbs, the scores identifying the degree of disability in each. Incoordination, interpreted as cerebellar in origin, is scored in the same way on either side of the bars representing pyramidal lesions. The thin black line scores the degree of disability due to a sensory deficit, visual defect, or both, originating in a cortical lesion. Each pattern is illustrated pictorially by the matchstick figure above the histogram. Case records of characteristic examples are given in the Appendix.

Graphic representation of the four clinical syndromes, although admittedly limiting, seems an acceptable way of describing and grading the physical disabilities due to individual neural lesions so that comparisons can be made between one patient and another. It also seems to be a succinct and readily communicated way of illustrating observations so that others can compare the data presented in this series with their own.

In the state of *decerebrate dementia* decerebrate reflexes are the principal response to stimulation. Initially there is tonic extension of the legs with extension or flexion of the arms, which, after many weeks, may give way to flexion of all four limbs, but more commonly to flexion of the arms and partial flexion of one leg. Semipurposive movement of a limb may develop on one side after many months. In the majority of cases there is no detectable intellectual function, but there may, ultimately, be some form of emotional response to the spoken word or gesture. Prolonged survival is uncommon, although occasional cases set memorable records. In the consecutive series not one was alive 10 years after injury, but since one patient in the selected series was still alive almost 10 years later, it has been assumed in figure 5.1 that perhaps 0.5 per cent of patients surviving post-traumatic amnesia or unconsciousness longer than a week might still be alive in states of demented decerebration as long as 10 years after injury. The probability that this is an overestimate is discussed with other evidence in chapter 14, concerned with the epidemiological aspects of this study.

In the *athetoid pseudobulbar* syndrome there is evidence of severe bilateral pyramidal damage with postural dystonia and often striking bradykinesia and fragmentary athetosis. In several patients there was a remarkable discrepancy between the severity of the physical disability and the relative preservation of personality and intellectual functions. This suggests that focal secondary infarction may contribute substantially to the residual deficit in this condition, rather than that the sole or principal cause is diffuse primary traumatic damage. The athetoid pseudobulbar pattern was seen in 16 patients (5 per cent) of the consecutive series. There were 20 cases amongst the 40 survivors of a month's coma in the selected series, and 12 amongst the 24 survivors of a month's coma in the consecutive series; that is 50 per cent in each.

In a commoner pattern of neural lesions the most striking feature was the evidence of associated cerebellar and pyramidal damage. This was invariably asymmetrical. Although the pathology is clearly not confined to the brain-stem, it is certain that this condition reflects the lesions found extensively throughout the brainstem by Tomlinson (1970), due either directly to trauma or secondary to compression from brain swelling or surface compression. The cerebellar component predominated more frequently than the pyramidal. For these reasons it seemed appropriate to call this the *brainstem cerebellar pattern*. It was encountered in 58 patients (20 per cent) of the consecutive series, and in 22 (34 per cent) of the combined selected series.

In the most frequently seen pattern of residual neural lesions there were signs of a pyramidal lesion on only one side. In the majority of cases these were minimal, consisting of slightly brisker tendon reflexes, a mild spasticity, often confined to the forearm pronators or quadriceps, and a plantar response that was extensor or less briskly flexor on one side. These signs were usually associated with some loss of facility for repetitive fine movements of an upper limb, or with a disturbance of gait typical of a unilateral pyramidal lesion. In addition there was often slightly defective balance, facial impassivity and a minor degree of dysarthria. This *hemiparetic* pattern was found in 115 cases (40 per cent) in the consecutive, and in only six cases (9 per cent) in the selected series. A dense hemiparesis was associated with the three preceding patterns of neural lesions except in six instances.

In the consecutive series 61 patients (21 per cent) had no detectable neural lesion, and 41 (14 per cent) with minor residual abnormal neural signs could not be assigned to any of these groups.

The question of the contribution made to these four patterns of residual neural damage by primary trauma and secondary infarction, the latter presumably due to brain swelling, surface compression, or cerebral perfusion failure, was examined by studying the evidence of deterioration recorded after admission to hospital. It was found that those patients whose level of responsiveness had deteriorated one grade or more after admission to hospital, as defined in table 5.1, or who had developed a new or worsening hemiparesis, accounted for two-thirds of the *brainstem cerebellar* group, for one-third of those with the *decerebrate dementia* and *athetoid pseudobulbar* syndromes, but for less than a quarter of the *hemiparetic*. The severity of the brainstem syndrome was greater amongst those who had deteriorated. Further evidence supporting the suggestion that the severity of the brain injury is closely related to these secondary factors rather than to primary traumatic damage becomes apparent when the incidence of skull fracture is examined in relation to duration of coma in table 5.2. It might be supposed

Table 5.2   Skull fracture in complicated and uncomplicated injuries related to duration of coma

Uncomplicated consecutive, coma less than 1 month	
Total number of patients	200
Number with skull fracture	122
Percentage with skull fracture	61%
Complicated consecutive, coma less than 1 month	
Total number of patients	67
Number with skull fracture	60
Percentage with skull fracture	90%
Uncomplicated selected, coma 1 month or longer	
Total number of patients	41
Number with skull fracture	20
Percentage with skull fracture	49%
Complicated selected, coma 1 month or longer	
Total number of patients	23
Number with skull fracture	18
Percentage with skull fracture	78%

that if traumatic brain damage, rather than secondary ischaemic infarction, were the principal determinant of the duration of coma, skull fracture would be seen more frequently in those with prolonged coma. In fact the reverse is the case in both complicated and uncomplicated injury.

The extent to which each of these four patterns of residual neural lesions was physically disabling in domestic, social and occupational spheres is examined in table 5.3. In assessing the overall degree of disability caused by these neural lesions only the highest score for any component of the pattern has been taken into account, and no distinction has been made between the degree of disability caused in domestic, social or occupational spheres of activity. It would appear that only amongst the younger patients is the athetoid pseudobulbar syndrome not severely disabling.

Brief decerebration due to surgically treatable lesions did not result in serious persisting disability. On the other hand, injuries complicated by surface brain compression or polar contusion and swelling requiring decompression were generally found to be associated with a greater prevalence of both abnormal neurological signs and some degree of persisting disability. Cortical sensory deficits and homonymous visual field defects persisted more often in complicated injuries.

An examination of the relationship between the side on which the head was struck and the side of the residual pyramidal lesion, or, if demonstrable in all four limbs, the side on which it was most marked, is made in table 5.4 and figure 5.2. In 134 cases the site of head impact was deduced from the site and

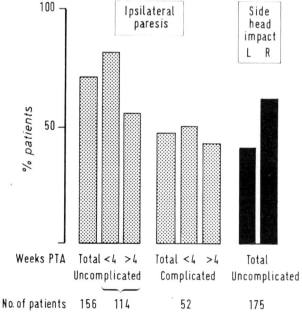

Figure 5.2 Relevance of the side of the head impact to the side of the hemiparesis, and to the length of the PTA defining the severity of the head injury on which selection of patients for inclusion in the study was based.

Table 5.3 Residual neurophysical disability associated with each of the four patterns of central neural lesions

	Decerebrate dementia		Athetoid pseudobulbar		Brainstem cerebellar		Hemiparetic		No abnormal neural signs		Unclassifiable	
Consecutive series (total 291 patients)												
Number and percentage	0		16	5%	58	20%	115	40%	61	21%	41	14%
Severely disabled or worse												
Uncomplicated injury			7 }	82%	9 }	24%	1 }	5%			2	
Complicated injury			6 }		5 }		5 }					
Moderately disabled or better												
Uncomplicated injury			3	18%	31 }	76%	79 }	95%	52		30 }	95%
Complicated injury					13 }		30 }		9		9 }	
Selected series (total 64 patients)												
Number and percentage	4	6%	32	50%	22	34%	6	9%				
Severely disabled or worse	4	100%	28	87%	9	41%	5	84%				
Moderately disabled or better			4	13%	13	59%	1	16%				

distribution of skull fractures as suggested by Lissner, Gurdjian and Webster (1949), Gurdjian, Webster and Lissner (1950) and Gurdjian and Webster (1958), and in a further 29 cases by the side of facial fracture. In the rest of the 175 patients the site of head impact could be identified certainly by contusions alone.

Table 5.4   Side of head impact and side of pyramidal lesion related to age and PTA in uncomplicated and complicated consecutive series of patients

	Side of pyramidal lesion and side of head impact							
	Ipsilateral				Contralateral			
	Uncomplicated		Complicated		Uncomplicated		Complicated	
Age at injury	<26	26+	<26	26+	<26	26+	<26	26+
Weeks PTA								
<4	52	40	4	8	12	10	4	9
4+	15	9	6	7	10	8	7	9
All ages								
Weeks PTA								
<4	92		12		22		13	
%	81%		49%		19%		51%	
4+	24		12		18		16	
%	57%		41%		43%		59%	
Total no. patients	116		23		40		29	
Percentage	75%		44%		25%		56%	

	Uncomplicated	Complicated
Weeks PTA		
<4	114	25
4+	42	27
Total no. patients	156	52

Total number of patients in consecutive series, 291. Total number of patients with side of head impact identified who had pyramidal lesions lateralised, 208.

It may be seen that in uncomplicated injury the less severe the head injury, assessed on the basis of length of post-traumatic amnesia, the higher the incidence of ipsilateral pyramidal lesions. In injury complicated by surface compression or brain penetration this evidence of 'contre-coup' brain damage is no longer apparent.

A cortical sensory deficit was not seen 10–24 years after injury except in association with readily demonstrable signs of a pyramidal lesion. This was not the case with homonymous field defects originating in hemisphere damage. These were occasionally seen on the same side with minimal evidence of a pyramidal lesion. It may be seen in table 5.5 that both these relatively uncommon residual signs were nevertheless more frequently found on the side of the head that had been struck in uncomplicated injury.

Table 5.5 Side of head impact and side of homonymous visual field defect and sensory deficit of hemispheric origin demonstrable at follow up in complicated and uncomplicated injury

	Visual field defect		Cortical sensory defect		Both	
	Right	Left	Right	Left	Right	Left
Uncomplicated injury*						
Right head impact	6	0	3	0	0	0
Left head impact	0	3	0	4	0	1
Complicated injury†						
Right head impact	2	5	1	0	1	3
Left head impact	2	2	2	1	3	1

* Fisher's test $P < 0.002$.
† Not significant.
Note: In 22 other patients with visual field defects and/or cortical sensory defects the head impact was either frontal, occipital or not possible to determine,
Total consecutive series of 291 patients.

Table 5.6 Incidence of dysphasia at the time of injury or in convalescence related to side of head impact

	Number of patients with dysphasia	
	Uncomplicated injury	Complicated injury
Right head impact	38	14
Left head impact	17	16

Total consecutive series of 291 patients.

The relationship between side of head impact and the incidence of dysphasia recorded in the hospital case notes during the acute period after injury or in convalescence is examined in table 5.6. Again, in injury uncomplicated by surface brain compression the close association between right-sided head impact and left cerebral hemisphere damage may be seen. The relative infrequency of persisting dysphasia demonstrable during the routine neurological examination is in striking contrast to this high incidence recorded shortly after injury. Nevertheless there was a permanent, although subtler, impairment of overall cognitive function demonstrable after right-sided head impact which was greater than that associated with left-sided impact. This was shown by a detailed psychometric assessment of 77 consecutive right-handed men from amongst all the patients with uncomplicated injuries in the consecutive series, who were followed up and tested between 10 and 20 years after their injuries. The results are described and discussed in the following chapter.

Discussion

This study provided a unique opportunity to examine, after the lapse of a substantial period of time, a large number of head-injured patients who were seen within the course of a year, and the majority within 6 months. These patients were unselected except by clearly defined criteria of the severity of the head injury. It had been stressed by Russell (1966) that there was a need to study an unselected series of patients with head injuries in order 'to get the feel of the clinical syndromes' which result from concussion. In a study, designed along similar lines, of an unselected series of ex-professional boxers re-examined 12–40 years after the end of their careers (Roberts, 1969), it had been the author's experience that there was a readily recognisable syndrome attributable to the cumulative effects of repeated minor concussion. In this present study of another large series of patients similarly seen in the course of a few months, it rapidly became apparent that there were four very different clinical syndromes attributable to damage to the central nervous system.

There have been a number of earlier reports of severely disabling post-traumatic syndromes which, it would seem, are highly selected variants of the four patterns of neural lesions described above. The best known of these are the states of 'traumatic apallia', first described by Kretschmer (1940), 'akinetic mutism' of Cairns, Oldfield, Pennybacker and Whitteridge (1941), the 'post-coma hypertonic stupor' of Fishgold and Mathis (1959), and the 'persistent vegetative state' of Jennett and Plum (1972). In the present investigation there were only two patients still alive at the time of the study and examined by the author in whom there was no response to stimulation identifiable as other than reflex. In these patients there was little more than decerebrate or decorticate posturing of the limbs together with eye movement occasionally taking on a semblance of purpose. Each patient was otherwise totally immobile and mute in the absence of stimulation, and without evidence of intellectual function. There was one other patient, aged eighteen when re-examined, who had been injured 9 years earlier. Three of her limbs responded to stimulation only by decerebrate posturing, yet she was capable of making some stereotyped movements of one arm which occasionally seemed purposive. In addition she was alert and able to evince pleasure and discomfort by giggling or crying in apparently appropriate response to simple spoken phrases or threatening gestures. She retained well-developed emotional responses of distress, anger and fear which were associated with exaggerated facial expressions. There was also no doubt that despite severely impaired visual acuity and a homonymous field defect she made attempts to fixate. There was no evidence at all of comprehension of the spoken word, but it was apparent that it was only the left arm with which she made semi-purposive movements, and also she was right-handed. It seemed virtually certain that her emotional responses to the spoken word were to the tone and simple affective connotation rather than to the content of what was said.

There were still signs of some minimal increase in the range of her responsiveness from year to year. Another man, aged nineteen at the time of his injury, remained, so far as could be judged from the information contained in the original case records, and thereafter from the detailed descriptions of his state in annual medico-legal reports, in an unchanging state of mindless mute and decerebrate akinesia for 3 years. At 7 years there was no alteration in his physical state but he was able to utter a poorly articulated 'Yes – no – hello' in response to questions. There was no evidence that these represented comprehension of the questions, or indeed any cerebral activity which might be regarded as sentient.

Despite the range of variation in the reflex and behavioural responses available to these four patients, it did not seem that the disturbance of neural function or the extent of the disability this caused differed materially, and there appeared much to be gained from considering them variants in degree of the same pattern of 'decerebrate dementia'. In support of this view there was the similar largely unchanging condition of 39 other patients who had survived for various periods longer than 3 months first in mesencephalic coma – as defined by Plum and Posner (1972) – and then in states of mindless decerebration until death. These are referred to again in chapter 12, where life expectancy is considered. There were many variants of the syndrome, but in all, the range of neural responsiveness was similar to that observed in these four survivors, and the long-term prognosis for both the virtually static clinical state and for survival, was identical.

Gerstenbrand (1967) and Vigouroux, Baurand, Choux and Guillermain (1972) describe the sequential progression from deep coma and tonic decerebration to states of persisting demented decerebration, with more or less marked evidence of consciousness and primitive motor automatisms. These authors distinguish between 'apallic deficit states' and *'pauci-relationnels'* states as sequelae of traumatic apallia, but it is not clear to what extent they would be prepared to consider the most severe, but not entirely unresponsive, variants as separately classifiable in terms of prognosis. Jennett and Plum (1972) are evidently of the opinion that 'the persistent vegetative state' excludes any response that is other than autonomic and reflex. They similarly fail to discuss in what way they consider the long-term prognosis is likely to be different for the decerebrate and 'mindless' patient, whose responsiveness is marginally greater, in that the reflex range includes primitive emotional expression and motor automatisms other than withdrawal.

In their review of a series of 190 patients admitted with severe disabilities to a rehabilitation unit, Cohadon, Hubert and Richter (1972) describe a pattern of lesions dominated by what they refer to as 'akinesia and axial hypertonus'. They encountered this in 23 patients. They are evidently describing, within months of severe brain injury, the condition found persisting years after their injuries in 38 patients examined for the present study, that is the pattern of 'central neural lesions' classified as the 'athetoid pseudobulbar' syndrome. It is also clear that in his 'apallic deficit state' Gerstenbrand (1967) is describing a similar condition in a number of instances. All these authors comment on the fact that where there is rapid improvement there may be little residual deficit in the course of many months. There were four children and three adolescents in the present series with minor forms of the syndrome. The remaining adult cases were all still profoundly disabled.

The 'mid-brain syndrome' of Kremer, Russell and Smyth (1947), and the cerebellar syndrome described as 'sequelae of traumatic lesions of upper brainstem and cerebellum' by Gerstenbrand, Lucking, Peters and Rothemund (1970), are evidently the same as the severe variant of the brainstem cerebellar pattern of lesions seen in the present study. Gerstenbrand and his colleagues found it in two-thirds of their series of 130 patients who had developed traumatic apallia after passing through an acute stage of 'mesencephalic coma', and in nearly all their cases these authors considered it attributable to compression of the upper brainstem and tentorial herniation. It is likely that a few of the cases described by Boller, Albert, Le May and Kertesz (1972), and attributed by them to traumatic brainstem damage because of the atrophy demonstrable here by air encephalography, were clinically similar. That aqueduct dilatation is invariably associated, or that it is only seen in this particular post-traumatic neural syndrome, as these authors suggest, is not the case. In their more recent study Peserico, Merli, Gerosa, Galligioni and Marin (1973) have shown that aqueduct enlargement after head injury is infrequent, and not consistently related to any post-traumatic neural syndrome. Indeed one of the most striking cases of post-traumatic dilatation of the aqueduct described by the latter authors appears to be associated with a severe athetoid pseudobulbar syndrome.

Two-thirds of the patients seen in the present study who were left with the more severe variants of the brainstem cerebellar pattern of lesions, had exhibited marked deterioration in their neurological state after admission to hospital. Their level of response to stimulation had declined one grade or more, they had developed a hemiparesis, or minimal limb weakness had progressed to severe paralysis.

The majority of the patients examined for this study were left with minimal signs of neural lesions, the most readily demonstrable of these being evidence of unilateral pyramidal injury. It seemed appropriate to classify these residual signs of brain injury together as the 'hemiparetic' pattern. It is clear that Maury and his colleagues, Miller and Stern, and Fahy and his associates, together with many other authors whose reports were cited in the review of the relevant literature (see chapter 2), have noted this as the commonest sequel of 'cerebral neural' damage found in survivors of severe, closed, acceleration head injury.

It would seem then that these four patterns of lesions and their variants are generally recognised by those who have examined large numbers of patients at long intervals after injury. The question arises as to whether these different clinical syndromes, which may persist indefinitely, reflect qualitative rather than quantitative differences in the pathological processes involved, and to what extent they can be assumed to be due to the same kind of damage as that seen in the brains of patients who die of their injuries. Although no pathological evidence was examined in the present study, a number of the long surviving cases of akinetic decerebration reported and discussed by Strich (1956, 1961) are included amongst the dead reviewed in a later chapter. To what extent the extensive cerebral white matter degeneration and brainstem lesions, which she described and attributed to shear strain primary trauma, contributed to the athetoid pseudobulbar or brainstem cerebellar lesions noted here, cannot be answered on the evidence available from this present study. It does seem highly probable, however, that the majority of the minimal hemiparetic and minor brainstem patterns of residual lesions found in patients who, relatively infrequently, had deteriorated after admission to hospital, were attributable to primary traumatic injury rather than to secondary infarction; the more so since there is a much closer association between the side of head impact and the side of the residual pyramidal lesion in the less severely disabled. It is certain that varying degrees of primary traumatic brainstem injury are a relatively constant finding after closed, uncomplicated head injury, as Tomlinson (1970) and Oppenheimer (1968) have shown. Whether these primary traumatic lesions, torn axons and arterioles, in brainstem and cerebral white matter, are often, or even solely, responsible for the syndrome of traumatic decerebration or its variants remains debatable. When decerebration is instantaneous, as Strich points out, it is difficult to conceive of any other explanation. According to Tomlinson, raised intracranial pressure causing brainstem displacement and distortion produces secondary haemorrhagic or ischaemic infarction in areas of the brainstem supplied by perforating arterioles, and this tends to obscure the lesser degrees of primary traumatic injury compatible with survival. In the view of Jellinger and Seitelberger (1970) it is the presence or absence of secondary brainstem lesions, and their specific pattern of distribution, which preferentially determines prognosis in states of 'protracted post-traumatic encephalopathy'. Tomlinson appears to agree with, or at least not to debate, this possibility, but he does not accept the view of these authors that all brainstem lesions in long-term survivors are secondary, or, for that matter, that long survival in states of decerebration is always due to secondary haemorrhage or ischaemic infarction of the brainstem. Jellinger and Seitelberger have confirmed, however, that secondary brainstem damage due to raised intracranial pressure and tentorial herniation is very common in the most severe closed head injuries, to which, after long survival, patients eventually succumb. That the occurrence of brain swelling is frequently the cause of raised intracranial pressure in these severe injuries is shown by the wedge-shaped areas of pressure necrosis in cingulate and hippocampal gyri. These Adams and Graham (1972) have identified as the hallmark of raised intracranial pressure. They are commonly found in cases where there has been no question of surface brain compression. The neurological status of two-thirds of the patients with the severe brainstem cerebellar syndrome, seen in the present study, had deteriorated after admission to hospital, suggesting, in the absence of surface compression, that brain swelling was the cause. In these cases it is reasonable to suppose that the residual neural syndrome was mainly due to secondary infarction attributable to conditions developing some time after the head injury. Conceivably, therefore, these were still amenable to treatment, particularly of raised intracranial pressure, had this been more readily available, for example, by the kind of controlled hyperventilation reviewed by Gordon (1972).

Patients who were left with the athetoid pseudobulbar syndrome deteriorated substantially less frequently after admission to hospital. As in the case of patients with persisting decerebrate dementia, the neurological state had declined a grade or more after admission in only one-third of cases.

Since, in the patients studied by Gerstenbrand and his colleagues, all those who developed the cerebellar syndrome survived, these authors were only able to infer pathological correlates by examining other cases who died whilst they were still apallic and decerebrate, and therefore without cerebellar signs. In these they found, as had Strich, and later, Jellinger and Seitelberger, asymmetrical, severe, microscopic and macroscopic damage in superior cerebellar peduncles, and cerebellar white matter. Their opinions differ as to the aetiology of these lesions, the latter authors and Gerstenbrand favouring oedema and secondary infarction due to brainstem compression rather than the shear strain mechanical forces proposed by Strich.

A point made by Gerstenbrand and his colleagues was that the development of this cerebellar pattern of injury implied a favourable prognosis as far as survival was concerned. They did not suggest, however, that this might be taken as evidence favouring different pathological processes to account for the two very different decerebrate apallic and brainstem cerebellar clinical syndromes, rather than just varying degrees of the same process.

The similarities between the athetoid pseudobulbar syndrome and many cases of congenital diplegia was apparent in the present study; they were also commented on by Maury and his associates, who observed them in patients treated in their rehabilitation unit. It was a remarkable feature of some of the cases seen in the present study that, despite profound, almost sloth-like, bradykinesia and spasticity of all four limbs, there was negligible impairment of balance, as is also characteristically the case in most cerebral diplegics. It seems possible, therefore, that cerebral perfusion failure, causing widespread ischaemic infarction, particularly of the basal ganglia, as described by Graham and Adams (1971a, b), may be more relevant here than infarction secondary to brainstem compression. The latter seems more commonly to be the process underlying severe forms of the brainstem cerebellar syndrome.

That the persistent athetoid pseudobulbar syndrome must sometimes be due to focal, ischaemic, secondary damage, and not to primary trauma, is apparent in the case of the six patients in the present study who, whilst profoundly disabled by their motor lesions, were relatively well-preserved intellectually, and were without severe personality disorders. The role of hypoxia in determining disability after severe closed head injury was examined by Price and Murray (1972), but without comment on the clinical, neurological disabilities of the surviving patients. Their view was that cerebral perfusion failure caused by impairment of cerebrovascular autoregulatory mechanisms, and due to a combination of hypoxia and raised intracranial pressure, was commonly associated with failure of social rehabilitation even in the long-term. The report by Solé-Llenas and Pons-Tortella (1974) on their angiographic studies of 67 severely head-injured patients, shows that ischaemic lesions due to perfusion failure at sites of cerebral contusion and also elsewhere throughout the brain, are often present in those who survive. It is not clear how often patients survive the extensive border zone ischaemic infarctions, due to the same mechanisms, described by Graham and Adams (1971 a, b), but it does seem reasonable to propose that this is likely to be the major pathological process responsible for the clinical state in a proportion of the patients surviving with the athetoid pseudobulbar syndrome and in those with variants of the pattern of decerebrate dementia. It is also highly probable that in these cases hypoxia occurred at or shortly after injury, when laryngeal reflexes were inadequate to prevent inhalation of blood and vomit. Amongst the patients unconscious longer than a month there is a smaller proportion with skull fractures than in the total series of patients with uncomplicated injuries. This is further evidence of the greater importance of secondary factors rather than of primary trauma in severe and persisting disability after closed head injury.

It is clear that there must be considerable overlap in the various pathological processes and that damage attributable to perfusion failure and brainstem compression often occurs together. If, nevertheless, it were possible to make an early distinction, either clinically or by modern techniques of medical measurement, between irremediable ischaemic infarction associated with cerebral perfusion failure at the time of injury, and that threatened later on by rising intracranial pressure and brainstem compression, the most distressing cases of decerebrate dementia and athetoid pseudobulbar disability might be avoided.

Assuming that these four persisting clinical syndromes do reflect major differences in the intensity of the underlying pathological processes, and that those due to primary trauma are more frequently the basis of the minor residual hemiparetic and brainstem cerebellar patterns, the question arises as to whether an examination of the mechanisms involved in primary traumatic brain injury might permit a more accurate prediction of the short- and long-term neural disabilities they cause.

If the patient described in the Edwin Smith surgical papyrus, and claimed by Breasted (1930) to be a case of contre-coup brain injury, really was one, then the observation that the site of head impact bears some relation to the side of limb paresis is at least 5000 years old. There have been repeated, and increasingly frequent, references to this association over the past 300 years. These have been supported by progressively more sophisticated and informed explanations based on theories of mechanics and the physical properties of the brain. Fallopius (1584) held that the force of the blow to one side of the head might be transmitted through the brain substance to the opposite side causing contusion, and Grima (1766) considered that the resistance of the skull opposite the side of the blow caused the shock passing through the brain to disrupt it there. Saucerotte (1769) felt that the undulatory movements of the skull transmitted through the liquid column of brain substance between the side of head impact and the opposite side were the cause of contre-coup injury. Sabauraut (1768) evidently held similar views, although he concluded that contre-coup lesions might occur anywhere in the brain regardless of the site of impact. As a result of his experimental observations with sand-filled skulls, Alquié (1865) considered that it was actual compression of brain against the opposite side of the skull which caused the contre-coup lesion. Variants of these mechanisms were proposed by Courville (1942, 1950), and by Lindenberg and Freytag (1960) on the basis of their pathological observations. These authors did not comment on any clinical correlations which they had observed or of which they were aware.

Serial electroencephalographic observations made by Dawson, Webster and Gurdjian (1951) provided confirmation, in those surviving their injuries, that in closed head injury the more severe damage was usually sustained by the temporal lobe opposite the side of impact. In a study of macroscopic surface contusions in a consecutive series of 151 fatal closed head injuries, Gurdjian, Webster and Arnkoff (1943) confirmed that wherever the head was struck, these were to be found, preferentially, in orbitofrontal and polar and lateral temporal areas. Courville (1958) states that almost invariably the most severely damaged areas are found opposite the side of head impact, and Spatz (1950) made a similar observation. More recent pathological evidence, both from accidental closed head injury and from experimental acceleration injury in primates, has been reported by Sano, Nakamura, Hirakawa, Masuzawa, Hashizume, Hayashi and Fujii (1967), Zülch (1969) and Ommaya, Grubb and Naumann (1971). These authors also draw attention to their observation that lateral, parietal and temporal blows cause maximum injury to the brain on the side opposite the point of impact, but that frontal impacts are likely to produce more severe macroscopic damage at the site of impact.

According to Holbourn, quoted by Strich (1961), the distribution of microscopic damage due to the internal shear strains which result from the violent rotational movements within brain tissue in closed head injury, although equal, is asymmetrical in the two hemispheres. This is due to the fact that the cerebral hemispheres are mirror images of each other and are rotated about different planes of symmetry. Strich (1956) had observed that pyramidal degeneration was characteristically asymmetrical in cases of severe head injury surviving for many months in states of decerebration, and she later (Strich, 1970) noted that traumatic demyelination was usually most marked in the pyramidal tract opposite the tear in the corpus callosum. Goldsmith

(1970) has reviewed theories of the mechanics of head injury and, with minor qualifications, concludes that Holbourn's shear strain hypotheses, proposed and elaborated in a series of papers (Holbourn, 1943, 1944, 1945) are likely to be correct. Oppenheimer (1968) suggested that the scattered microglial clusters he found in the brains of a number of patients who had died after closed head injuries of varying severity were at sites of axonal tearing due to the mechanical forces described by Holbourn. Using a modified version of the same staining technique, Clark (1974) has since shown that the intensity of these microglial clusters is greater in the corpus callosum on the side of the head struck and in the internal capsule and brainstem opposite.

Despite this substantial body of information on the subject of contre-coup brain injury there has been little systematic study of the relationship between the site of impact to the head and the clinical evidence of neural dysfunction in closed head injury.

In the present investigation a relatively close relationship has been shown in the case of the less severe injuries. The disabilities caused by this contre-coup brain damage in the form of pareses, impaired cortical sensory functions and visual field defects are slight in the long-term. The more important relationship between side of head impact and cognitive deficits will be examined in the next chapter.

It would seem therefore that, in all probability, the four patterns of neural lesions observed in this study do reflect differing pathologies, albeit overlapping ones, rather than simply varying degrees of the same pathology, and that the long-term outlook for the disabilities each produces closely and predictably reflects the nature of the underlying pathological process.

6 Patterns of Personality Disorder and Intellectual and Memory Deficits

Clinical Assessment

In making this clinical assessment of personality change and impairment of intellectual functions, information was obtained from three sources, as described in the method of investigation (pp. 25–26). Briefly, these were the observations of the patient himself; of a relative, usually parent or spouse and in many cases both; and also the clinical assessment made of the patient when he was interviewed. As with patterns of persisting central neural lesions, but often a little less clear-cut than these, there were features of personality change and impaired intellectual function which tended to occur together.

The most frequently recurring complex was one in which the most striking features were euphoria and disinhibition, together with irritability and a defective memory. It was possible to assess the degree to which each of these features of personality change and impaired intellectual function was disabling in the spheres of domestic, social and occupational life by using the same method of scoring as for the assessment of physical disability due to neural lesions. This is illustrated in table 6.1. In the same way, bar histograms

Table 6.1   Assessment of mental disability

Grade	Score	Intellectual impairment and/or level of consciousness	Personality change
Decerebrate dementia	5		
Purposive or semi-purposive response to stimulation	4.5		
Total dependence	4	Inaccessibly demented or delirious or stuperose	Inaccessibly psychotic
	3.5	Demented or confused but accessible	Psychotic but accessible
Profound disability	3	Comprehending and/or obeying or dysmnesic or dysphasic	Psychiatric illness and/or other personality disorder

Precluding normal domestic *or* social
or occupational life

Table continued overleaf

Table 6.1 — *continued*

Grade	Score	Intellectual impair- ment and/or level of consciousness	Personality change
Severe disability	2.5	Dysphasia, memory defect or other intellectual impairment	Personality change
		Limiting substantially household management, domestic harmony, social intercourse *or* employment	
Moderate disability	2	As above	As above
		Causing *difficulties* in marriage, social adjustment *or* job	
Slight disability	1.5	As above	As above
		Causing *inconvenience* only in domestic, social *or* occupational spheres	
Minimal disability	1	As above	As above
		Awareness of slight forgetfulness, loss for a word, irritability having *minimal effect* on home, job *or* socially	
Negligible disability	0.5	As above	As above
		Apparent only to examiner or relative and of *no significance* in domestic, social *or* occupational spheres	
No disability	0		

provided a convenient method of studying which features of the personality change or intellectual impairment were, or were not, associated, and to what extent each was disabling. The eight principal patterns are illustrated as 'mental disability profiles' in figure 6.1. As with patterns of central neural disability, each was assigned a descriptive title, coined with the intention of drawing attention to characteristic features of the disorder and, at the same time, to the sites of focal brain injury these reflect. There are precedents for attempting to describe post-traumatic personality disorders in this way, and, however inadequate, this does provide a shorthand method of identification which will avoid unnecessary repetition. Broca himself, in describing 'the great limbic lobes' (Broca, 1878) suggested that they represented 'the brutish' part of the cerebral hemispheres. This, taken together with recent evidence, to be cited later, which indicates that this area is especially vulnerable in closed acceleration injury, seems to provide some justification for the use of the term in describing characteristic features of one of the commonest patterns of personality disorder observed in this study.

In scoring these 'profiles' a number of features of the personality change which might better have been considered separately, were summated. Numbers were small. For the purposes of this study it seemed reasonable to accept as reflecting damage to similar areas in frontal lobes, personality change which included euphoria, disinhibition, irresponsibility and childishness, a blunting of emotional responsiveness towards children or spouse, the loss of former drive and initiative, as well as apathy and anergia. Since hyperkinesia is also an occasional sequel of frontal leucotomy (Rylander, 1939; Reitmann, 1946; Partridge, 1950), the three patients whose energy output and activities were unexpectedly and favourable increased after their injuries were also assumed to have had 'frontal' personality change. Similarly anxiety, whether specifically phobic or a general increase in apprehensiveness in social situations or at work, and also when associated with a depressive illness, has been included in the same bar of the histogram.

There were 50 patients in the consecutive series with the most frequently encountered pattern of *frontolimbic dementia* (figure 6.1(a)). Here scores for disability due to frontal personality change and intellectual impairment tended to be the same as scores for the intense, associated irritability. In other words, if euphoria, disinhibition, irresponsibility or anergia prevented or hampered employment, then aggressive and irritable outbursts were liable to do the same, or to make domestic life and normal social contact insupportable or difficult to a similar extent. In a proportion of cases scores for 'irritability' were much higher, and in many patients this feature of the traumatic alteration of personality, rather than the associated dementia, euphoria, disinhibition or apathy, was the principal cause of domestic misery. Outbursts of violent and ungovernable rage were the most severely disabling form assumed by this 'release' of irritability and again, it was this rather than the dementia which led to the long-term commitment of four patients (figure 6.1(b)) to psychiatric institutions. It was striking how often the main target and victim of ill-tempered and violent outbursts was the spouse, an observation recently also made by Behrman (1975) on a small number of head-injured patients.

The majority of those with severe physical disability due to athetoid pseudobulbar and brainstem patterns of neural lesions displayed this type of 'mental disability'. It varied in degree, tending to parallel, but almost always exceeding the degree of disability due to impaired 'central neural' physical functions. This was not invariably so however. Severe neural disability was found in six patients who, although profoundly forgetful, had relatively well-preserved personalities and other intellectual functions. This is further evidence which suggests, contrary to some recent assumptions of Ommaya

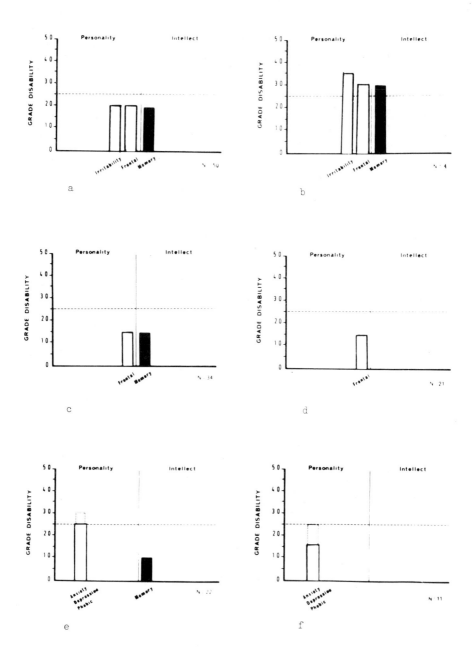

Figure 6.1   Mental disability profiles. (a, b) Frontolimbic dementia; (c) frontal dysmnesia; (d) frontal; (e, f) dysmnesic inadequacy and phobic imbalance; (g) traumatic dysmnesia; (h) isolated dysphasia; (i) frontal and irritable; (j) irritable and dysmnesic; (k), (l) two examples of full mental disability profiles showing personality changes and cognitive deficits for two cases (S265, S35) from the consecutive series.

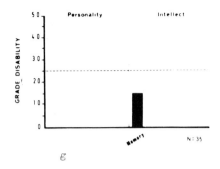

g

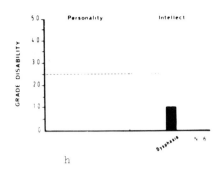

h

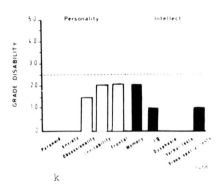

k

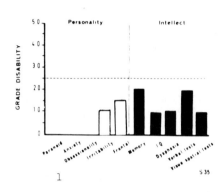

l

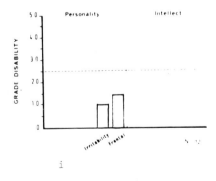

i

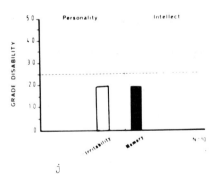

j

and Gennarelli (1974), that focal secondary infarction may contribute substantially, and to a greater extent than diffuse primary traumatic damage, to the residual deficits.

In the consecutive series there were 21 patients, the larger proportion of them under the age of thirty-five at the time of injury, in whom there was only evidence of a mild *frontal* personality change (figure 6.1 (d)). There was no release of irritability and no impairment of intellect or memory, so far as could be judged clinically or from the account given by the relatives. None was severely disabled by neural lesions.

The commoner pattern of *frontal dysmnesia* (figure 6.1 (c)) was mostly seen in those individuals whose injuries had occurred between the ages of twenty-six and thirty-five years. It was found in 34 patients and consisted of euphoria, disinhibition, childishness, or loss of initiative and drive, associated with slight impairment of day-to-day memory, but without irritability. As with the preceding pattern, there was seldom other than minimal neural disability, and this, despite the fact that post-traumatic amnesia had often been prolonged. Except in the very young there had been neither prolonged decerebration nor prolonged coma.

There were seven patients who were less anxious and prone to worry after their head injury and who were more outgoing and sociable than they had been before. Three of them were more energetic and effective. Five of these patients had a mild but persisting impairment of day-to-day memory. It is difficult to explain this personality change, reminiscent of the most successful effects of selective inferomedial frontal leucotomy in chronic tension states, except as a sequel to traumatic lesions in similar areas of the frontal lobes. Despite the fact that, in most cases, this improvement in personality was at the expense of some minor forgetfulness, it can hardly be described as a disabling outcome of the injury. On the other hand, since personality change was being assessed, it seemed reasonable to make an arbitrary score of 1.5 on the disability scale in the case of these patients. This permits their inclusion in later discussions of the relevance of focal brain damage to the outcome of closed head injuries. The disability caused by these patterns of mental change is examined in table 6.2 in relation to age at the time of injury and to the severity of the injury as judged by duration of post-traumatic amnesia.

The combination of a mild defect of memory and disabling anxiety was a common sequel of injury after the age of thirty-five. The anxiety often seemed to be reactive to vestibular disturbance, or to memory impairment or both. In many patients apprehension that they might lose their balance and fall had evidently served to worsen and then to perpetuate disability due to the disturbance of equilibrium caused by vestibular damage. The resulting disorder, best described perhaps as *phobic imbalance*, limited the patients' activities to varying degrees. At its worst the individual was virtually confined to the house by agoraphobia. The intensity of this form of disability tended to decline over the course of 2 years or so (as indicated in the histograms) but there was often considerable restriction of normal activities which persisted,

Table 6.2 Patterns of mental disorder related to age at injury and severity of disability and PTA

	Grade disability			
	Slight or worse (1.5+)		Minimal (1)	
	Weeks PTA			
	<4	>4	<4	>4
Frontolimbic dementia (N=50)				
Age at injury { 26+	3	17	6	1
Age at injury { <26	2	14	6	1
Frontal dysmnesia (N=34)				
Age at injury { 26+	4	6	6	3
Age at injury { <26	0	3	9	3
Frontal, frontal and irritable or irritable alone (N=39)				
Age at injury { 26+	9	2	13	2
Age at injury { <26	0	3	8	2
Dysmnesia alone (N=35)				
Age at injury { 26+	0	4	7	0
Age at injury { <26	8	4	7	5
Phobic imbalance or dysmnesic inadequacy (N=22)				
Age at injury { 26+	14			
Age at injury { <26	8			
Anxiety alone (N=11)				
Age at injury { 26+	3			
Age at injury { <26	8			

Total consecutive series of 291 patients (142 < 26 at injury, 149 26+ at injury).

especially amongst older patients, and this without any evidence of a neural lesion.

A similar association, anxiety and a defective memory for day-to-day events, seemed appropriately designated *dysmnesic inadequacy*. Instead of phobic imbalance there was an inability to cope with normal domestic, social and occupational responsibilities which in part at least, seemed to be determined by doubts as to intellectual incompetence, imagined or real but elaborated. Invariably there was heavy dependence upon the spouse. Both of these conditions were often associated with depressive symptomatology, and in a number of instances the accident was followed for many years by depressive illnesses. So far as could be judged in retrospect, there were few whose premorbid personalities had clearly predisposed them to recurrent anxiety depressions, although this was certainly the case in some instances. In general, younger patients with persisting anxiety as the sole manifestation of their personality change had no neural disabilities, and most showed no evidence and made no complaint of defective memory either. These personality disorders in which anxiety predominated were seen in 33 patients (figure 6.1 (e, f)), 22 with and 11 without defective day-to-day memory.

A persisting impairment of day-to-day memory without evidence of personality change and without any suggestion of impaired verbal or visuospatial functions, in so far as this could be assessed clinically, was one of the most frequently encountered mental sequelae of these head injuries. This isolated *traumatic dysmnesia* was found in 35 patients amongst the consecutive series (figure 6.1 (g)). In the majority it caused only slight disability. If neural lesions were associated with defective memory there was usually also a frontal personality change, or marked irritability, or both.

This frequently encountered disturbance of memory functions seems certain to reflect damage on both sides of the brain in the medial parts of the temporal lobes, that is in both hippocampal regions and in their different pathways via fornices to mamillary bodies. In contrast, evidence of persisting verbal or visuospatial functions, reflecting focal unilateral hemisphere damage, was rare in the absence of dementia or severe neural disability. There were only six patients who were still having difficulty expressing themselves verbally over 10 years later, yet who were not either severely demented or neurologically disabled (figure 6.1 (h)). The fluent jargon with which one of these patients answered every question was quite unlike the hesitancy in naming and finding the appropriate word characteristic of most patients with persisting dysphasic difficulties. On the other hand it was reminiscent of some focal dysphasias seen in cerebrovascular disease. This patient was in his fifties when he was injured. Secondary infarction due to failure of left middle cerebral artery perfusion seemed the most probable cause. The infrequency with which persisting *dysphasia* was encountered contrasted with the relatively high incidence of varying degrees of dysphasia recorded in the hospital notes for short periods after the injury (table 5.6) and recalled by many patients and their relatives.

Only two patients admitted to continuing difficulty in recognising familiar faces and finding their way about familiar places. As with dysphasia many others vividly recalled such difficulties, due to impairment of visuospatial function, lasting several weeks or months following their return home after the injury. No relationship could be established between this latter disorder and the side the head that had been struck, or with the post-traumatic agoraphobia.

There were only 12 patients who had a persisting slight to moderate *frontal* personality change, and who were disabled by *irritability* to a comparable extent, yet were not also forgetful (figure 6.1 (i)). There were only 10 patients with persisting *irritability* and *forgetfulness* who did not show some evidence of euphoria, disinhibition, loss of affect or other frontal personality disturbance (figure 6.1 (j)).

Paranoid delusional symptoms had evidently been experienced transiently during the period of post-traumatic confusion by many patients. Even more frequent was the experience, admitted by almost a third of the patients, of an intense self-consciousness associated with ideas of reference and suspicion, which often lasted a year or more, and occasionally persisted to a lesser degree indefinitely. Persisting paranoid psychoses were uncommon and almost invariably associated with dementia, although the degree of dementia was not always severe. In the consecutive series those patients who developed *schizophreniform psychoses* are detailed briefly in table 6.3. There were four patients who, as they recovered from their injuries, developed progressively worsening delusional psychoses. Two of these patients became progressively more demented, one in association with poorly controlled epilepsy and the other with alcoholism. The other two patients became increasingly forgetful but their psychotic illness was substantially more disabling than their intellectual impairment. There were two further patients moderately demented by what it seemed reasonable to conclude were the effects of normal brain ageing superimposed upon traumatic brain damage, who were also paranoid and subject to ill-systematised delusions. Another patient demented progressively due to intractable epilepsy 8 years after his injury, having ideas of reference, revelatory experiences and delusions that he was the godhead. In none was there a family history of schizophrenia. One patient in the selected series was considered to be *paraphrenic*. His symptoms were not in evidence prior to injury. Both his mother and his sister were chronic schizophrenic inmates of psychiatric hospitals. The only two patients with schizophrenia-like psychoses who were not demented did not develop their illnesses until many years after injury.

A number of more or less demented patients were liable to respond intermittently with paranoid behaviour and ideation in certain situations which varied with the individual concerned. These were not a constant feature of their behaviour but rather, a non-specific concomitant of their traumatic dementias.

In addition there were four patients who, over long periods, had displayed and were still evincing *pathological jealousy*. In two cases this was associated with impotence and in one with increased libido and performance. The remaining patient was a married woman whose husband described pathological jealousy in association with increased libido which gradually declined in intensity but was still in evidence 12 years after the injury.

Depressive illness was distinguished from reactive depressive symptomatology in making assessments of disability only by disability scores. There was no patient with a depressive illness which did not include an element of anxiety and, as explained above, both depression and anxiety were scored in the same bar of the mental disability histogram. A total of 16 patients had developed depressive illnesses since their injuries. In eight cases this followed directly upon the injury; six of these patients subsequently suffered from recurrent depressions, one alternating with hypomanic swings and all with the features of endogenous illnesses. In four cases endogenous depressions had been delayed for 1.5–2 years, apparently developing as the frontal personality change regressed. In these 12 patients, that is 4 per cent of the consecutive

Table 6.3   Prevalence of 'schizophreniform' psychoses in patients examined in consecutive series

Case number and sex	Age at injury	Age at onset	Age examined	Duration PTA	Diagnosis and associated neural disability
Case 1,* Male S41	25	42	46	10 days	Paraphrenia or schizoaffective psychosis with ideas of influence in a cyclothyme 17 years after injury. Residual peripheral facial palsy the only neural lesion.
Case 2, Male S94	32	32	47	4 weeks	Moderate traumatic frontolimbic dementia gradually worsening with paranoid poorly systematised delusions of reference for past 8 years. Severe optic chiasmal injury, otherwise asymmetry of tendon reflexes the only sign of neural lesions elsewhere. Temporal lobe epilepsy before and after.
Case 3, Male C82	35	35½	49	2 weeks	Florid paranoid psychosis a few months after injury. Progressive dementia thereafter with paranoid ideas of influence and reference. Poorly controlled generalised convulsions at the rate of 15 or more a year. Less frequent epileptic attacks preceded and caused the injury. Brainstem cerebellar pattern of neural lesions.
Case 4, Male S36	44	44	65	5 weeks	Recurrent endogenous depressions treated with ECT before and since, the former hypochondriacal and the latter with paranoid ideas of reference. Slowly progressive paranoid dementia for past 6 years. Mild brainstem cerebellar pattern.
Case 5,* Male S101	46	55	60	2 weeks	A dozen or more episodes lasting several weeks at a time, the first 9 years after injury, of depression with paranoid ideas of influence and reference. Mild brainstem cerebellar syndrome.

Table 6.3 — *continued*

Case number and sex	Age at injury	Age at onset	Age examined	Duration PTA	Diagnosis and associated neural disability
Case 6, Male S18	46	46	65	Permanent	Traumatic dementia slowly worsening since injury with paranoid ideas of reference and ill-systematised delusions of persecution. Heavy drinker before, spree-drinking malnourished alcoholic after injury. A few post-traumatic generalised convulsions controlled by anticonvulsants. Brainstem cerebellar pattern.
Case 7, Male S212	55	55	67	4 weeks	Post-traumatic delirium with paranoid delusions of persecution second day after injury, and thereafter moderate dementia with paranoid ideas of influence and reference. Mild brainstem cerebellar pattern.
Case 8, Female S279	55	55	68	6 weeks	Paranoid ideas of reference and mildly demented since. Unclassifiable pattern of neural lesions causing negligible disabilities.
Case 9, Male C9	20	28	33	4 months	Severe athetoid pseudobulbar pattern of neural lesions with frontolimbic dementia gradually continuing to improve till 8 years after injury. Then, with increasing frequency of post-traumatic generalised convulsions, progressive personality change with ideas of influence and paranoid ideas of reference. A second head injury during a fit 12 years after the first complicated by an acute subdural haemotoma was succeeded by further deterioration both mental and neural suggesting a communicating hydrocephalus. Questionable hypopituitarism.

* The only patients not demented

series, it seemed certain that the head injury had been responsible for the illness. The remaining four patients did not develop their depressions until several years after injury and in these cases the injury was apparently incidental.

There were three cases of *suicide* amongst the total consecutive series of 468 patients. Calculating on the basis of 7000 successful suicides annually in this country, and adjusting for the proportion at risk in the 10–24 years since their injury, it may be approximately estimated that this is three times the expected number. In addition there were three patients who made suicidal gestures. Considering the appalling physical and intellectual disabilities endured by many of these patients for months or years before tolerable recovery was achieved, and suffered indefinitely by some patients, it is perhaps surprising that there were in fact so few suicides. It may be that the leucotomising effects of the injury, an almost invariable accompaniment of the more severe brain damage, were of some relevance here.

Obsessional symptomatology in the form of excessive checking and tidiness seemed to have been determined equally by constitutional predisposition and by post-traumatic intellectual impairment. There were only two patients whose obsessional disabilities were sufficiently intense to be regarded as typical of obsessive compulsive neuroses. In both cases these had developed only after the injury, but there had been indications of pathological obsessionalism in both of them before this. In neither was there any other personality change, intellectual impairment or neural lesions to suggest a traumatic organic substrate for the illness. Two other patients without evidence of brain injury were pathologically obsessional after their injuries.

Analysis of the relationship between the side of head impact and the foregoing clinical evidence of personality change and defective memory failed to reveal any consistent association. Similarly no association was found between personality disorder and the lateralisation of visual field defects and pyramidal lesions.

Psychometric Tests of Cognitive Function

The following results refer only to the data obtained testing 77 right-handed males, whose injuries were uncomplicated, from amongst the consecutive series of patients. Initially it had been intended to test every patient in both the unselected consecutive, and in the more severely injured, selected series. In the event the time taken by each patient to complete the full battery of psychometric tests made some selection necessary. In addition to the exclusion of patients who were left-handed, a number of females were not tested since it is held that dominance for verbal functions may be less consistently established in one hemisphere amongst females. It soon became apparent that few data in a form suitable for statistical analysis were likely to be forthcoming from testing the more seriously demented who could attempt and complete few of the tests. A higher proportion of these came from the consecutive series of patients whose head injuries had been complicated by surface compression. The same problem arose with testing those in the selected series who had survived the more severe head injuries. Thus, although a total of 199 patients from the consecutive and 37 from the combined selected series underwent some part of these tests of cognitive function, it was decided to abandon a detailed analysis except in the case of the 77 consecutive male dextrals. A more limited attempt to examine the significance of the results of one verbal and one visuospatial subtest, together with a score for overall intelligence, was made by converting scores to the 'disability' grades used in the clinical assessment and studying them in relation to the eight mental disability profiles. These results will be presented later.

The tests used to examine various cognitive functions in these 77 right-handed males have been described in the chapter on the design of the investigations. The data derived from this limited study were analysed using a multivariate analysis of variance computer programme described by Baughan (1973). Separate values were computed for main effects and interactions. Relationships were examined between test scores and four principal variables: the age of the patient at the time of the accident, the age at the time of the follow-up examination, the duration of post-traumatic amnesia and the state of neurological responsiveness in the first 24 hours after admission to hospital. The distribution of the 77 male dextrals in relation to the variables examined is set out in table 6.4, and their mean ages in table 6.5. The relationship between these and the side and site of head impact in the injury was also studied. Only significant results are tabulated.

From tables 6.6, 6.7 and 6.8 it can be seen that amongst those who were struck on the right side of the head, scores in all verbal and visuospatial tests were significantly lower than scores amongst those whose head impact was on the left. There were also significant interactions between side and site of head impact. Those struck on the left frontal and right parietal regions of the head had major deficits in visuospatial skills. In table 6.9 it can be seen that there were no significant differences in IQ between those struck on the left and right sides of the head. Cognitive impairment as examined in these tests was not significantly related to the duration of the post-traumatic amnesia, the state of neurological responsiveness on the day of admission to hospital, or to the age at which the injury was sustained. Amongst patients struck on the right side of the head, however, there was a decline in performance with increasing age both at the time of injury and of testing, but the differences do not reach conventional levels of significance. Similarly, although scores were lower amongst those struck on the right side whose post-traumatic amnesia had lasted from 2 to 3 weeks or longer than a month, there was no consistent decline in the scores for the cognitive functions tested with longer-lasting amnesia.

This analysis did not include an examination of the duration of either decerebration or coma. It is possible that, had it done so, differences in test

Table 6.4   Distribution of 77 dextral male patients in relation to variables examined

| | Side of head impact | |
	Left (N=36)	Right (N=41)
Site of impact		
Frontal	21	24
Lateral	6	7
Parietal/occipital	9	10
Duration of post-traumatic amnesia		
1 to < 2 weeks	4	7
2 to < 3 weeks	15	16
3 to < 4 weeks	15	14
4 weeks or longer	2	4
Neurological status on first day		
Decerebrate	3	6
Purposive	18	18
Confused	15	17
Age at injury		
5–15 years	3	7
16–35 years	27	25
36 years and older	6	9
Age tested		
16–35 years	12	15
36–55 years	20	19
56–65 years	4	7

Table 6.5   Mean age of patients (in years) at testing

| | Side of head impact | | | |
| | Left | | Right | |
Site of impact	Means	S.D.	Means	S.D.
Frontal	42.7	8.8	37.6	10.2
Lateral	45.4	9.2	36.6	15.6
Parietal/occipital	39.5	13.3	49.1	12.3

scores might have emerged that could be related to these two measures of severity of the injury. The numbers were too small, however, in the case of the patients who had been decerebrate but were still able to complete the full battery of tests, and since there is a close correlation between duration of unconsciousness and length of post-traumatic amnesia it is probable that significant differences might have been demonstrable only for prolonged coma as for prolonged amnesia.

Table 6.6   Mean scores in verbal tests in left and right head impact groups of patients

	Left		Right		P	
	Means	S.D.	Means	S.D.	Sig.*	I†
Object naming latency and site of impact						
Frontal	59.10	7.26	60.42	7.34		
Lateral	58.80	7.13	62.54	8.90	0.05	0.05
Parietal/occipital	54.98	5.29	64.86	5.59		
Object naming (%) and duration PTA						
1 to < 2 weeks	86.53	3.32	82.40	9.60		
2 to < 3 weeks	88.95	10.39	77.44	12.18	0.05	0.05
3 to < 4 weeks	82.45	13.62	86.80	9.38		
4 weeks or longer	90.38	1.92	72.11	14.48		
Object naming (%) and neural status 1st day						
Decerebrate	89.74	1.81	75.63	13.26		
Purposive	89.17	10.68	78.84	13.46	0.05	
Confused	81.58	12.21	85.10	8.53		
Object naming (%) and age at injury						
5–15 years	96.15	3.14	76.36	3.20		
16–35 years	84.97	12.28	83.71	14.32	0.01	
36 years and older	85.89	7.90	76.91	6.77		
Object naming (%) and age tested						
16–35 years	88.84	14.85	81.79	10.64		
36–55 years	84.29	9.38	82.62	14.20	0.05	
56–65 years	86.53	7.92	74.71	5.74		

* Significance for main effect of side of impact.
† Significance for interaction between side and site of impact.

Table 6.7   Verbal memory and learning test scores

	Left		Right		P*
	Means	S.D.	Means	S.D.	
Delayed story recall and age at injury					
5–15 years	6.83	2.01	5.71	3.08	
16–35 years	5.81	2.85	4.64	3.17	0.05
36 years and older	7.41	3.23	3.83	1.87	
Digits recall and age at injury					
5–15 years	7.00	0.81	5.00	0.92	
16–35 years	6.40	1.06	6.28	1.11	0.01
36 years and older	6.50	0.95	5.66	1.24	
Immediate story recall and age tested					
16–35 years	8.00	3.62	6.93	3.59	
36–55 years	8.42	2.58	6.68	2.90	0.025
56–65 years	8.87	2.32	5.14	1.72	

Table continued overleaf

Table 6.7 — *continued*

| | Side of head impact | | | | |
| | Left | | Right | | |
	Means	S.D.	Means	S.D.	P*
Digits recall and age tested					
16–35 years	6.58	1.11	5.86	1.30	
36–55 years	6.40	0.96	6.10	1.07	0.05
56–65 years	6.50	1.11	5.57	1.29	
Paired associate learning and site of impact					
Frontal	11.38	3.43	10.25	3.79	
Lateral	12.78	2.17	9.85	2.98	0.025
Parietal/occipital	12.83	3.04	10.25	4.62	
Immediate story recall and site of impact					
Frontal	7.59	3.27	6.58	2.78	
Lateral	9.14	1.84	7.14	3.54	0.01
Parietal/occipital	9.27	2.19	5.90	3.32	
Delayed story recall and site of impact					
Frontal	5.38	3.14	4.33	2.39	
Lateral	6.85	2.29	5.71	3.26	0.05
Parietal/occipital	7.22	2.17	4.65	3.75	
Delayed story recall and duration PTA					
1 to less than 2 weeks	7.37	3.47	6.35	2.04	
2 to less than 3 weeks	6.40	2.68	3.93	2.38	0.05
3 to less than 4 weeks	5.63	2.93	5.25	3.57	
4 weeks or longer	6.00	2.50	2.37	1.55	
Immediate story recall and neural status 1st day					
Decerebrate	8.83	2.01	6.41	2.00	
Purposive	8.50	3.15	6.66	3.98	0.05
Confused	8.03	2.84	6.38	2.16	
Delayed story recall and neural status 1st day					
Decerebrate	7.83	0.94	2.41	1.30	
Purposive	6.11	3.03	5.38	3.45	0.01
Confused	5.90	2.95	4.64	2.41	
Immediate story recall and age at injury					
5–15 years	9.33	1.31	7.42	3.33	
16–35 years	7.88	3.05	6.80	3.19	0.01
36 years and older	9.83	2.44	5.00	1.81	

* Level of significance for main effect of side of impact.

Table 6.8   Non-verbal test scores

	Left Means	Left S.D.	Right Means	Right S.D.	P Sig.*	P I†	P Site‡
WAIS designs immediate recall and site impact							
Frontal	6.90	3.49	8.20	2.64			
Lateral	9.42	1.59	8.57	3.59	0.025		
Parietal/occipital	8.11	2.92	4.80	3.28			
WAIS designs delayed recall and site impact							
Frontal	4.42	3.59	5.29	2.90			
Lateral	5.57	3.06	5.42	2.96	0.025		
Parietal/occipital	7.00	3.49	3.85	2.50			
WAIS designs delayed recall and age at injury							
5–15 years	9.66	2.86	6.14	2.23			
16–35 years	4.44	3.60	5.16	3.48	0.025	0.025	0.05
36 years and older	6.83	1.95	2.00	2.35			
Block design and site impact							
Frontal	9.90	2.75	11.29	3.27			
Lateral	11.85	3.35	11.71	2.71	0.01	0.001	0.025
Parietal/occipital	12.55	2.11	4.20	4.40			
Lattice maze and site impact							
Frontal	0.63	0.21	0.67	0.19			
Lateral	0.76	0.15	0.62	0.28	0.025	0.025	
Parietal/occipital	0.85	0.11	0.54	0.23			
Lattice maze raw scores and duration PTA							
1 to less than 2 weeks	11.00	1.42	8.57	3.00			
2 to less than 3 weeks	9.20	3.72	6.00	3.02	0.025		
3 to less than 4 weeks	9.20	3.83	7.57	4.59			
4 weeks or longer	9.00	1.00	5.25	2.28			
Lattice maze raw scores and neural status 1st day							
Decerebrate	9.66	1.24	7.00	3.26			
Purposive	9.66	2.78	6.50	4.36	0.025		
Confused	9.00	4.48	7.29	3.15			
Lattice maze raw scores and age at injury							
5–15 years	11.66	0.47	9.14	2.74			
16–35 years	8.62	3.59	7.00	3.67	0.001		
36 years and older	11.66	2.56	4.80	3.63			
Lattice maze and age tested							
16–35 years	0.74	0.16	0.70	0.17			
36–55 years	0.68	0.24	0.65	0.19	0.05		
56–65 years	0.76	0.04	0.44	0.31			

Table continued overleaf

Table 6.8 — *continued*

	Side of head impact				*P*		
	Left		Right				
	Means	S.D.	Means	S.D.	Sig.*	I†	Site‡
Lattice maze raw scores and age tested							
16–35 years	9.41	3.12	8.20	2.76			
36–55 years	9.15	4.01	6.84	4.09	0.01		
56–65 years	10.50	1.11	4.29	3.28			

* Level of significance for main effect of side of impact.
† Level of significance for interaction between side and site of impact.
‡ Level of significance for main effect of site of impact.

Table 6.9　IQ results

	Side of head impact			
	Left		Right	
	Means	S.D.	Means	S.D.
Progressive matrices: percentile, ranking, converted to IQ				
Frontal	91.19	23.70	93.62	25.56
Lateral	107.57	16.70	99.28	20.27
Parietal/occipital	99.88	11.38	80.30	41.71
Mill Hill vocabulary				
Frontal	83.61	29.54	83.54	27.86
Lateral	91.00	39.12	90.28	12.18
Parietal/occipital	95.11	12.44	87.90	9.61

Disability in Terms of Psychometric Cognitive Test Scores

In order to utilise at least a proportion of the data collected in testing intellectual function in the remaining patients, many of them the more severely brain-damaged who could not attempt or complete the full battery of subtests, a table was designed to convert the scores for one verbal and one non-verbal test to 'disability grades'. A similar conversion was made for the full scale percentile of the verbal and performance IQ scores. Disability grades were assigned arbitrarily to various ranges of test scores after their scatter amongst all the patients tested had been noted. These are given in table 6.10. The two tests used were the speed of object naming and the lattice maze test for the verbal and non-verbal subtests.

In table 6.11 it can be seen that patients with uncomplicated injuries tested with the lattice maze had significantly lower disability grades when the head impact had been on the right than when it had been on the left. This relationship between side of head impact and disability score can no longer be

Table 6.10   Psychometry test scores converted to disability grades

	Disability score	Disability grade
IQ percentiles		
70 or less	2	Moderate
80 or less	1	Slight
>80	0	None
Object naming (mean latency in milliseconds)		
4 and longer	2.5	Severe
3–3.9	2	Moderate
1.6–2.9	1	Slight
1.5 or less	0	None
Lattice maze (number attempted correct = raw scores)		
0–3	2.5	Severe
4	2	Moderate
5–7	1	Slight
8 or more	0	None

Table 6.11   Visuospatial test scores converted to disability grades and related to side of head impact

	Disability score*			Totals
	0	1	2+	
Number of patients with head impact on				
Right	42	23	24	89
Left	47	12	9	68

	Injury					
	Uncomplicated†			Complicated		
	Disability scores					
	0	1	2+	0	1	2+
Number of patients with head impact on						
Right	35	19	20	7	4	4
Left	40	8	5	7	4	4

Total combined series tested: 216 of 331 patients.
* Sig. $\chi_2^2 = 7.89$; $P < 0.025$
† Sig. $\chi_2^2 = 10.63$; $P < 0.005$.

SEVERE ACCIDENTAL HEAD INJURY

Table 6.12 Verbal and visuospatial cognitive tests and IQ converted to disability grades and related to duration of PTA

| | Disability grade | Weeks PTA | | |
		1–2	3–4	5+
Verbal test (speed of object naming)				
Number of patients	None	72	25	37
Percentage		65%	53%	61%
	Slight	31	17	13
	Moderate			
	or worse	9	5	6
		8%	11%	11%
Totals tested		112	47	56
Visuospatial test (lattice maze)*				
Number of patients	None	66	23	18
Percentage		60%	51%	40%
	Slight	22	10	12
		22%	22%	23%
	Moderate			
	or worse	21	12	15
		18%	27%	33%
Totals tested		109	45	45
IQ Full-scale percentile				
Number of patients	None	63	28	26
Percentage		57%	60%	38%
	Slight	36	14	22
	Moderate			
	or worse	12	5	10
		10%	11%	17%
Totals tested		111	47	58

Total combined series tested: 216 of 331 patients.
* Sig., $\chi_2^2 = 5.31$; $P < 0.025$.

shown for the verbal subtest as it could in the case of the 77 dextrals with relatively less severe head injuries. Table 6.12 shows that where post-traumatic amnesia has been prolonged the visuospatial test results are significantly poorer, assessed by these disability gradings. There is a similar trend in IQ percentile scores, but again not in the case of the verbal test. It seems likely that these observations are explained by the inclusion of the more severely brain-injured patients in these assessments of intellectual function. As in the case of the relationship between side of head impact and lateralisation of pyramidal lesions, described in an earlier chapter, in the more severe injuries and also in injury complicated by surface brain compression, the evidence of contre-coup brain damage tends to be obscured. When these subtler effects of primary traumatic brain injury are lost there are grosser overall defects of cognitive function which show a closer relationship to the severity of the injury as measured by the duration of the post-traumatic amnesia.

The Relationship between Occupational State and Mental and Physical Neural Disability

The relative contributions of the mental and physical after-effects of brain damage in these injuries to the success or failure of occupational rehabilitation are examined in table 6.13. It may be seen that within each age group there are substantially more patients whose occupational status has declined because of impaired personality or intellectual function than because of their neural lesions. This is as true of the skilled manual as of the clerical worker, and only in unskilled manual workers is physical disability as liable to be associated with a decline in job status as mental disorder. In social classes 1 and 2 there were 32 individuals whose occupational status had declined and of these only 22 had a degree of central neural physical disability graded slight or worse in contrast to 30 with similarly graded mental disability. In social classes 3 and 4 there were respectively 41 and 51 individuals whose occupational status had declined, 27 and 33 with neurophysical disability graded as slight or worse compared with 38 and 46 with similar degrees of mental disability. Only amongst the 35 unskilled manual workers whose job status had fallen were there almost as many with similar grades of neurophysical and mental disability, that is 29 and 31 respectively. These differences are significant.

Examining the data in a different way it was found that amongst the consecutive series of 214 patients whose injuries were uncomplicated there were 86 who had experienced a permanent decline in job status following their accidents. In 48 individuals the score for mental disability was higher than the score for central neural disability, in 18 the scores for neural were higher than for mental disability, and in 21 cases the two disability scores were the same. In other words, where disability scores were not identical, in nearly two-thirds of those with a lower occupational status, personality change or intellectual impairment seemed more likely to have been responsible than neural disability, and in only one-third of cases did neurophysical rather than mental disability appear more likely to be the cause.

In this analysis women who, prior to injury, had some form of employment in addition to looking after a household were reckoned to have suffered a decline in occupational status if they did not subsequently return to a job. The ability to look after a household and cope with the shopping unassisted, despite some mental or physical disability, has been assessed as 'unchanged' so far as occupational state is concerned. The social class and occupational status of children injured before commencing secondary education were assumed to have been those of the parents and comparisons were made with these in the assessment of changes. It could not be shown that a decline in occupational status was related to the side the head was struck in the injury.

Table 6.13   Occupational status before and after injury related to neurophysical disability

	Total declined	Grade central neurophysical disability			
		0-0.5	1-2	2.5-3	3.5+
Social classes 1 and 2 (professional and/or university, managerial, teacher, nurse, lab technician)					
Same		16	3		
Decline	32	10	10	10	2
Rise		2	1		
Social class 3 (skilled manual, clerical)					
Same		34	13	1	
Decline	41	14	10	13	4
Rise		3		1	
Social class 4 (semi-skilled manual)					
Same		40	6	1	
Decline	51	18	15	14	4
Rise		5			
Social class 5 (unskilled manual)					
Same		31	11		
Decline	35	6	16	11	2
Rise		3	1		
Social classes 1 and 2					
Same		10	9		
Decline	32	2	16	12	2
Rise		2	1		
Social class 3					
Same		18	28	2	
Decline	41	3	17	17	4
Rise		2	2		
Social class 4					
Same		25	21	1	
Decline	51	5	23	20	3
Rise		2	3		
Social class 5					
Same		12	27	3	
Decline	35	4	8	21	2
Rise		2	2		

Total combined series of 331 patients.

Discussion

It must be admitted that in presenting these patterns of disordered personality and intellectual function there has been considerable over-simplification of the mental after-effects of closed acceleration head injury. There is much, nevertheless, that seems in accord with the observations of others who have sought for an explanation of post-traumatic personality disorders in focal brain damage. Individual interests, however, have usually confined comments to only a few of the syndromes described here.

In penetrating brain wounds of the frontal lobes Kleist (1934) drew attention to the predominantly psychomotor, 'lack of drive' and cognitive deficits following convexity lesions, which were in striking contrast to the emotional and behavioural disorders associated with orbito-frontal injury.

Kretschmer (1949) distinguished between two types of post-traumatic personality change which he suggested were due to 'orbito-frontal' and 'hypophyseal-diencephalic' damage. In the first he appears to be describing the usually accepted characteristics of frontal lobe injuries, that is 'loss of normal sense of tact and social restraint, poor emotional control and euphoria'. In the second he notes 'the release of sexual instinctual behaviour and oral activity, with hyperkinesia and aggressive rage', and their frequent association with disorders of hypothalamic and pituitary function. It would seem that the most frequently occurring syndrome noted in the present study, and referred to as *frontolimbic dementia*, combines elements of the two described by Kretschmer, and that in the second of these he is observing an early, transitional stage, through which many of the patients seen in the present study had also passed.

In a short-term follow-up study and examination of a constellation of post-traumatic symptoms which included pathological irritability, affective disorders, memory impairment, changes in sexual potency, vertigo and headache, Lechner (1958) singled out contusion of one or both temporal lobes as its basis. The evidence he put forward was mainly electroencephalographic, but in support of his suggestion he referred to the well-established experimental animal work of Papez (1937), Kluver and Bucy (1939), Bard and Mountcastle (1948), and the case of a patient treated with bitemporal lobectomies reported by Terzian and Dalle Ore (1955).

Russell (1932, 1934, 1935, 1948), Russell and Nathan (1946) and Russell and Smith (1961) have drawn attention to the selective vulnerability in closed head injury of systems subserving registration and recall of on-going events. Russell was the first person to point out that this is illustrated by the close relationship between the duration of post-traumatic amnesia, the severity of the injury, and the subsequent mental and neural disability. In a more recent experimental study in primates subjected to violent rotational head movement, Ommaya and Gennarelli (1974) have shown that the macroscopic evidence of shear strain forces is most marked at the junction between the white and grey matter in the medial temporal and orbito-frontal areas of the brain (figure 6.2).

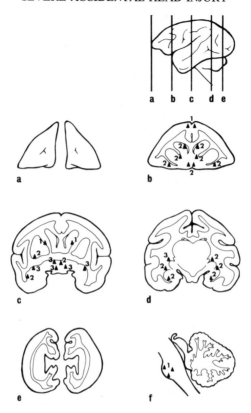

Figure 6.2　The distribution and intensity of microscopic shear strain damage found in the brains of 12 squirrel monkeys subjected to experimental concussive head injury by rotational head movement sufficiently violent to induce coma. (Redrawn from Ommaya and Gennarelli, 1974, with permission.)

Solid triangles (▲) indicate sites of petechial haemmorhage. The numbers indicate the frequency of occurrence of haemmorhages at each site as follows: 1, less than 50 per cent; 2, 50–75 per cent; 3, 75–90 per cent.

In the earlier-mentioned clinical study of post-traumatic encephalopathy in professional boxers examined many years after the end of their careers, Roberts (1969) found that, within each age group, the prevalence of forgetfulness was higher amongst those who had done the most boxing. The pathological basis for this latter cumulative effect of repeated minor brain injury has since been reported by Corsellis, Bruton and Freeman-Browne (1973). In the majority of the brains of 16 ex-boxers they found intense neurofibrillary degeneration in the hippocampus, together with severe atrophy of the forniceal afferent tracts to the mamillary bodies. The mamillary bodies were themselves the site of local injury as well as of trans-synaptic atrophy. These changes in the brain of one boxer are well illustrated by

Corsellis (1975) (figures 6.3 and 6.4). Such changes were most marked in the brains of the boxers who, in life, had been the most forgetful, and these were also the boxers who had done the most boxing.

In their careful study of the pathological effects of raised intracranial pressure due either to brain swelling or to surface brain compression, in closed head injury, Adams and Graham (1972) describe the invariable wedge-shaped infarcts they found in hippocampal and cingulate gyri adjacent to the

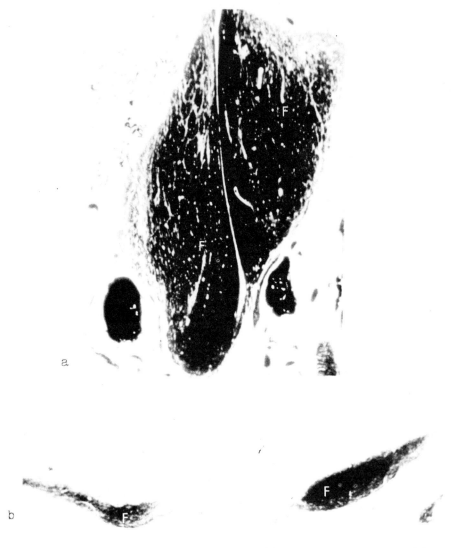

Figure 6.3 Coronal sections of the fornices of (a) a normal elderly man, (b) a punchdrunk dysmnesic ex-boxer of similar age. Photographed at the same magnification. (From Corsellis, 1975, with permission.)

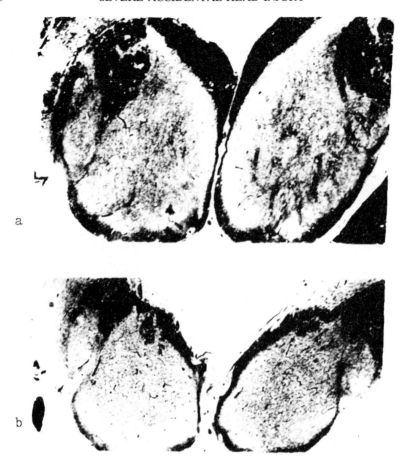

Figure 6.4   Coronal sections of the mamillary bodies of (a) a normal elderly man, (b) a
punchdrunk dysmnesic ex-boxer of similar age. Photographed at the same
magnification. (From Corsellis, 1975, with permission.)

tentorium and falx. These they attributed to pressure necrosis, which was
usually associated with focal haemorrhages, both due to brain herniation.

   Courville (1942, 1950, 1958), Gurdjian, Webster and Arnkoff (1943), and
Lindenberg and Freytag (1957, 1960) have drawn attention to the orbito-
frontal and temporal contusions which are so highly characteristic a feature of
severe closed head injury, whatever the site of head impact.

   Severe injury to the orbito-frontal white matter will destroy the fronto-
septal tracts identified by Nauta (1964) and Johnson, Rosvold and Mishkin
(1968). Severe injury to the medial areas of the temporal lobes will interrupt
the major sensory afferent projections from the cerebral cortex demonstrated
by Powell (1973). These dual systems converge on the hypothalamus, the first
directly from the orbito-frontal cortex, and the second via tracts within the

cingulate gyrus and from the entorhinal cortex via the hippocampus and the forniceal-mamillary projection. Extensive damage in these two regions must in effect disconnect the hypothalamus from the perceptual brain.

In the light of this evidence it would seem reasonable to propose that in the severest, closed, acceleration head injuries compatible with survival, whatever the extent and distribution of primary traumatic or secondary brain damage, it is to be found maximally in orbito-frontal and medial temporal areas, and the hypothalamus is likely to be virtually deafferented of cortical connections.

Recovery, if it occurs, does so in an orderly, sequential manner which Gerstenbrand (1967) has described in some detail. Coma and tonic decerebration give way to increasing alertness, and primitive motor automatisms, reminiscent of the early stages of neonatal development, provide a background to increasingly complex activity as cortical influences are restored. The first emotional responses to reveal themselves are invariably anxiety and fear, followed by irritability and rage. These, like the primitive motor behaviour, are progressively refined as cortical influences are restored and recovery continues. Depending upon the extent of irreparable neural damage in these subcortical sensory and motor pathways, the process of recovery may cease at any stage, leaving stereotyped patterns of defective neural, emotional and cognitive function, frozen as it were, at various stages in the course of recovery. In the severest injuries there are neural deficits of the decerebrate, athetoid pseudobulbar and brainstem patterns. More frequently there is incomplete cortical control of emotional behaviour characterised by frontal disinhibition and euphoria, the release of irritability and memory impairment.

Where the injury has been relatively less severe, or has occurred in childhood, adolescence or early adult life when there is probably a greater capacity for the restoration of disordered cerebral functions, the patient is often left with a personality change characterised by mild euphoria or disinhibition together with slight impairment of day-to-day memory, and this without the release of irritability. In rare instances this type of personality change actually constitutes an improvement. A few patients become less anxious and tense and are more sociable and energetic than they were before, as Storey (1967) and Logue, Durward, Pratt, Piercy and Nixon (1968) found in patients who had sustained cerebral damage due to haemorrhage from anterior cerebral aneurysms, and as Fahy, Irving and Millac (1967) noted after severe head injury.

According to the experimental evidence of Ommaya and Gennarelli (1974) and the pathological evidence of Adams and Graham (1972), damage due to shear strains and also to infarction secondary to raised intracranial pressure or brain compression is greater in medial temporal than in orbito-frontal areas. It follows that the subcortical system subserving the release of anger is either less vulnerable, despite greater damage, than that which inhibits frontal personality change, or is more readily restored to functional normality.

It is not clear what relationship exists between the post-traumatic irritability which seems comprehensible in psychodynamic terms, and the lesser variants of the uninhibited rage reactions which must be determined by focal injury in periamygdaloid areas of the temporal lobes. There are certainly neuronal centres in the posterior hypothalamus which are concerned with the experience and expression of anger in men. An extensive literature, reviewed by Sweet, Ervin and Mark (1969), and referred to by Zieman and King (1958), and also by Sano, Ishijima and Ohye (1962), Sano, Yoshioka, Ogashiwa, Ishijima and Ohye (1966), Narabayashi and Uno (1966) and Burzaco and Gutiérrez Gomez (1968), amongst a number of neurosurgeons practising 'sedative psychosurgery', describes an interdependent subcortical complex of neuronal masses and tracts capable of modification by tumours, surgery and trauma. It seems that discrete lesions at specific sites within the general periamygdaloid area are more likely to reduce irritability and aggression than injuries elsewhere. The more extensive the damage the more likely it is that there will be a lessening of the inhibitory mechanisms.

On the clinical evidence of the present study there can be little doubt that in the most severely brain-damaged cases the terrifying rages exhibited by many patients are organically determined. There must be declining degrees of this organically determined post-traumatic phenomenon which, at its least severe, may be completely indistinguishable from reactive irritability. It appears that irritability in the absence of frontal brain damage and memory defect is less likely to be explained on the basis of 'limbic' lesions after a single severe head injury. On the other hand, the association of irritability and defective memory without disinhibition and euphoria was a common sequel to repeated minor head injury in the ex-professional boxers studied earlier by the author (Roberts, 1969). As may be seen in table 6.14, with increasing occupational

Table 6.14   Defective memory and personality deterioration related to age and occupational exposure in random sample of 224 ex-professional boxers examined 10–30 years after retirement from the ring

| Age examined: | | 50+ | | | 49–30 | | |
Years as pro. boxer:		10+	9–6	5–3	10+	9–6	5–3
Totals	179	28	26	18	18	35	54
Number complaining							
of poor memory	50	13	12	3	7	7	8
Percentage*		46%	46%	17%	39%	20%	15%
Relative's account							
Totals	122	20	17	11	15	22	37
Numbers observed							
with poor memory	22	9	6	2	3	2	0
Percentage		45%	35%	18%	20%	9%	0
Numbers observed with							
personality change	30	7	9	2	4	5	3
Percentage		35%	53%	18%	27%	23%	8%

*$P < 0.02$.

exposure there was a trend towards an increasing prevalence of forgetfulness and a personality change dominated by irritability in each age group, although numbers were too small to satisfy conventional tests of significance, except in the case of memory impairment.

A similar association of irritability and memory defect was found in a selected series of eight retired steeplechase jockeys considered by Corsellis and Roberts (1975) and also, independently, by a number of other neurologists (Corsellis, 1976) to be suffering from a similar chronic traumatic encephalopathy due to repeated, relatively minor head injuries. Euphoria or disinhibition were seldom a feature of the encephalopathy in boxers or steeplechase jockeys.

To explain both these observations and those of the present study, it is tentatively proposed that they are a further illustration of the cumulative effect of repeated microscopic trauma in medial temporal areas and of the relatively greater resistance of the orbito-frontal white matter to shear strain injury in minor concussion.

This question of the extent to which there may be an organic basis for post-traumatic irritability was considered in some detail by Lishman (1968, 1973). His own studies concerned a series of patients with penetrating brain injuries due to gunshot wounds, who were followed up by questionnaire up to 5 years after injury. There appeared to be little relationship between the amount of focal brain damage, judged by the extent and depth of brain penetration, nor, for that matter, between the severity of diffuse injury, judged by the length of post-traumatic amnesia, and symptoms of impaired concentration, anxiety, depression and irritability. These were commonly associated with somatic complaints of headache, dizziness, fatigue and sensitivity to noise. In other words this constellation of post-traumatic 'neurotic' symptoms did not seem explicable on the basis of organic brain damage. In a later lucid review of the psychiatric sequelae of head injuries, including closed injuries, Lishman (1973) refers in some detail to the observations of Kretschmer (1940) noted above, and to the two important papers of Hooper, McGregor and Nathan (1945), and Black, Jeffries, Blumer, Wellner and Walker (1969). In these the authors had commented on irritability and rage reactions which were a highly characteristic sequel of severe closed head injuries in both adults and children. These did not appear to be neurotic reactions. Similar observations were made in a series of patients with severe closed head injuries studied by Kremer (1944).

There is clearly a major distinction to be drawn between discrete focal brain injury due to missile penetration, which is usually confined to one cerebral hemisphere, and the predominantly orbito-frontal and medial temporal damage on both sides of the brain typical of closed acceleration injury. Conclusions drawn from a study of missile brain injury, with respect to personality and intellectual functions at least, cannot necessarily be extrapolated to severe, closed head injury.

In contrast to these patterns of residual personality change and memory deficit, the two patterns designated *phobic imbalance* and *dysmnesic inad-*

equacy were infrequently associated with evidence of central neural lesions. They occurred with increasing frequency amongst those who were older than thirty-five at the time of injury. Anxiety, usually in the form of a phobic disinclination to leave the house and apparently due, in part at least, to impaired equilibrium, or to a less specific combination of anxiety and depression with feelings of inadequacy and inability to cope with previous responsibilities in occupational, social or domestic spheres, tended to be severely disabling, often for as long as 2 or 3 years. Pratt and McKenzie (1958) drew attention to the frequent tendency for phobic anxiety to perpetuate organically determined vestibular disorders, and Roberts (1964) noted the common association of serious organic illness with the onset of the first panic attack heralding a chronic agoraphobic state. More recently Hinoki (1971) seems to have confirmed by 'adrenalin loading' tests that vestibular disorders are demonstrably highly sensitive to the normal autonomic concomitants of anxiety and in so doing he provided at least one explanation of a traumatic 'neurotic' reaction in terms of genuine exaggeration of vestibular dysfunction. It is the author's impression that, in general, this perpetuation of organic imbalance by phobic anxiety is underestimated after head injury. The phenomenon is often attributed, misguidedly, to financial considerations when questions of compensation arise. In this study, disability due to these symptoms tended to decline over the first year or two, but often there was persisting limitation of activities and a failure to return to normal levels of employment or to assume normal domestic responsibilities and social life. The situation is remarkably reminiscent of the so-called post-concussional state commonly seen, but usually only for a limited period, after comparatively minor head injuries.

It might reasonably be proposed that the two conditions do have a similar pathological basis in damage to memory-forming pathways or to central or peripheral vestibular symptoms or both. In the older patient, and almost certainly also in the constitutionally predisposed, there develops a self-perpetuating anxiety response which is not seen in patients protected by the leucotomising effects of more severe head injuries.

In passing, it may be said that in less than a dozen cases in the entire consecutive series did it seem either likely or possible that questions of compensation had served to perpetuate mental or physical disability. In contrast, there were two patients who had recently sustained a second, but minor, injury. Following their serious head injuries 10 and 12 years previously, neither had behaved in such a way as to suggest that they had dramatised their transient disabilities, and yet both were clearly doing so for gain when reviewed within months of their minor injuries. On the other hand it was repeatedly apparent that, in the face of abundant evidence to the contrary, patients and relatives were prepared to underestimate the severity not only of mental disorders but even of very obvious physical disability, and to tolerate the consequences. Both of these observations would appear to support at least some of the views expressed by Miller (1961 *a*, *b*, 1966) on the subject of malingering for gain after injury, which is prevalent with a frequency inversely proportional to the severity of the injury and its consequences.

In an exhaustive review of schizophrenia-like psychosis associated with organic disorders, Davison and Bagley (1969) discuss the question of cerebral trauma. They suggest that in the single case it is rarely possible to be certain that cerebral trauma has been an aetiological factor in the subsequent development of a schizophreniform psychosis and they refer to a review of the German literature between 1900 and 1950 by Elsässer and Grünewald (1953). Applying strict criteria these authors concluded that there had only been 26 cases reported in which a causal relationship was probable. Moreover they held that, to be relevant, the brain damage must be severe and its temporal connection with the psychosis obvious; in other words that symptoms must be seen to have developed progressively since the head injury or out of its sequelae rather than incidentally after a long delay. In making the point that the most satisfactory method of establishing the entity of post-traumatic schizophreniform psychosis was by following an unselected series of head-injured patients over a long period, Davison and Bagley tabulated eight detailed reports culled from the literature where this had been attempted. These show an incidence of schizophrenia varying between 9.8 per cent and 0.4 per cent during periods of observation which ranged from 3 months to 20 years. According to these authors the expectation of developing schizophrenia in the general population is 0.8 per cent over a 25-year risk period in patients aged between fifteen and forty years, so that the incidence in the reports they cite suggests a threefold increase over the expected. They draw attention to the fact that Hillbom (1951) is one of the few authors who has provided details of the age structure of his brain-damaged population of war-wounded. The expected prevalence of schizophrenia in his 415 cases was two and the actual number observed was eleven.

In the present study, amongst the 291 survivors examined from the consecutive series there were only two who developed schizophrenia-like psychoses and yet who were not also demented. It is probable that both of these were basically affective illnesses. More important, symptoms of the psychoses did not develop until 9 and 17 years after injuries which, in both cases, were relatively less severe than those sustained by the majority. It would seem unwise therefore to assume that the head injury was in any way relevant in either case. The psychotic symptomatology displayed by the remaining seven patients might be more aptly described as *paranoid dementia* rather than post-traumatic schizophreniform psychosis.

The frequency of suicides after head injury has been the subject of comment by a number of authors. In his review of war-wounded examined up to 20 years after wounding, Hillbom (1960) noted a substantial excess even over the unusually high levels of suicide found in the general Finnish population. In the present study three successful suicides is a threefold excess over the expected incidence in the general population in the period under review and in addition there were three other patients who had attempted suicide without success.

Turning now to the results of the psychometric tests of cognitive function, some of which have already been briefly reported by Smith (1974), it appears that even in closed head injury there may be a relationship between the side the head is struck and the degree and character of the subsequent impairment of intellectual functions. Focal cognitive deficits after brain-penetrating missile injury were studied in great detail by Newcombe (1969), but there has been no previous report designed to examine the relationship of cognitive deficits to side of skull impact in closed head injuries.

Since the 77 consecutive right-handed males were all able to complete the full series of psychometric tests to which they were subjected, it follows that, in general, these were the subjects with the less severe intellectual impairment and lesser degrees of brain injury. They were also all patients whose head injuries had been uncomplicated by surface compression or brain penetration. In other words these patients were amongst those with evidence of pyramidal lesions, if they were present at all, on the same side as the head had been struck. It was perhaps surprising to find that visuospatial functions tested, as well as verbal, were relatively more impaired in those who were struck on the right side of the head, and the fact that visuospatial functions were not more impaired in those who were struck on the left needs an explanation.

It has been pointed out by Teuber (1962) and Lishman (1968) that not only verbal but also overall intellectual function assessed by psychometric tests is particularly vulnerable to left hemisphere damage by penetrating missile injury. Piercy (1964) commented on the same finding reported by McFie (1960) in a series of patients with a variety of neoplastic and other lesions confined to one or other cerebral hemisphere. It is probable as well that although the visual tests used in this study were sensitive to impairment of right visuospatial functions, they were not sufficiently sensitive to demonstrate the minor residual disabilities that the more complex tasks advocated by Teuber (1969) might have elicited. As Milner (1969) has also indicated, it may be that many visual memory tests are susceptible to verbal labelling and Zangwill (1960) has pointed out that certain visuospatial deficits can be associated with language disorders.

Cortical contusions underlying linear fractures are a well-recognised but normally minor complication of severe closed head injury. The question arises as to whether the poorer performance in tests of visuospatial function amongst those who were struck on the right side of the head was due to this mechanism. The fact that there was no striking impairment of verbal function observed which could be attributed to brain injury underlying ipsilateral fractures would seem to make this explanation a little unlikely. In all previous studies of closed head injury the relevance of side of impact to impairment of intellectual function has been neglected, with the single exception, that is, of a study reported by Heilmann, Saffran and Geschwind (1971) of a small number of patients, mostly alcoholics, with post-traumatic dysphasia. They noted, as in this study, that dysphasia was commonly associated with right-sided impact, although they also found that it was demonstrable, at least for the short period in which their patients were followed up, when the impact was to the skull overlying the left temporoparietal region. It is probable that in these latter cases cortical contusions underlying fractures had been the cause. The fact that similar observations were not made in the present study suggests that this mechanism may often cause only transient disturbance of function in contrast to the more permanent deficits attributable to the more severe contre-coup injuries.

In passing it may be noted that these subtle defects in intellectual function – still demonstrable by psychometric testing in the present study more than 10 years after a single severe closed head injury – did not appear to cause significant disability. On the basis of this evidence, however, it would seem that the side of head impact might be relevant in explaining some of the more elusive components of the shorter-lasting post-concussional syndrome, for example, complaints of difficulty in concentrating, and might repay further study.

The failure to demonstrate any relationship between the psychometric test results and the severity of the injury, when this was assessed on the basis of neurological responsiveness in the first 24 hours, needs explanation. Failure to consider the duration of decerebration or coma has probably caused their significance to be underestimated. However, Robertson and Pollard (1968) and Richardson (1963) also noted that decerebration in children and adolescents was not invariably associated with severe persistent intellectual impairment. Norrman and Svahn (1961) found that the initial state of neurological responsiveness correlated only with performance in a three-choice reaction-time task amongst the tests of cognitive function they used. In a more recent study Bond (1975) failed to show a decline in scores in the Wechsler Adult Intelligence Test with increasing post-traumatic amnesia, except where this had been prolonged. Amongst the 77 male dextrals who completed the full battery of tests a similar observation was made in the present study only in the case of individuals whose injuries had resulted in right-sided head impact. In the case of the majority of the more severely injured patients who were only able to complete some of the subtests, it was shown that increasing post-traumatic amnesia did result in a greater proportion of lower scores in the lattice maze test and possibly also in percentile IQ scores, but not in the test of speed of naming. On the other hand there were many patients who had suffered prolonged post-traumatic amnesia yet scored well on all these tests of cognitive function. Evidently the factors determining performance in tests of cognitive function after closed head injury are multiple and complex, and it would seem unwise to assume that any of the indirect measures of severity of the injury commonly used are likely to be more than inconstantly associated with performance in routine psychometric tests.

It was unfortunate that in this study limitations of time prevented the inclusion of a choice reaction-time task. This is so particularly since clinically slowness of thought was a striking characteristic of many of the patients examined. Lacking an explanation for this, the author initially recorded the phenomenon in every patient in whom it was observed as 'obsessionally slow mentation', leaving for later consideration the question of how far it was a reflection of constitutional obsessionalism and how far of post-traumatic psychomotor retardation. By the end of the study it was clear that both contributed to it, but in many cases it was still difficult to determine which was the more relevant factor amongst patients whose coma had lasted for less than a month. Over half of these individuals had some associated difficulty with day-to-day memory and a third had minor frontal personality changes.

In those most seriously injured there was certainly often a profound slowness and 'stickiness' of thought, as well as of movement, aptly referred to by Maury as 'intellectual viscosity'. It is more than likely that in the 'sub-cortical dementias' described by Albert, Feldman and Willis (1974) this phenomenon was being observed. In patients with progressive supranuclear ophthalmoplegia, extrapyramidal disease and thalamic lesions associated with tumours and vascular disease, these authors appear to be describing this clinical phenomenon in its severest form. Others have since demonstrated the same disorder in its less obvious form by formal psychometric techniques. Using a simple and choice reaction time task Miller (1970) was able to show that there was a reduction in the speed of 'processing information' amongst a series of patients who had sustained severe closed head injuries. It seems likely that this was the same disturbance of intellectual function found lasting only transiently in patients after minor concussive injuries by Gronwall and Wrightson (1974) using a timed serial addition test. This reduction in the 'speed of thinking' and the striking bradykinesia shown by most of the patients with the athetoid pseudobulbar syndrome in the present study, and the syndrome of akinetic mutism, are possibly related phenomena varying in degree.

Whether this reflects disordered function in reticular activating nuclei and their connections, and hence arousal mechanisms, as suggested by Albert and his colleagues, cannot be answered by any of the evidence presented here. The experimental models of the apallic syndrome studied by Dolce and Fromm (1972) in cats illustrate that, although the midline cerebral activating systems are frequently involved, a variety of lesions can be made in cerebral hemispheres, corpus callosum and brainstem which produce similar hypokinetic clinical states. Stimulating electrodes in pallidum and thalamus have been shown by Hassler, Dalle Ore, Diekmann, Bricolo and Dolce (1969) to cause arousal in patients with traumatic apallia. It is reasonable to assume that there is a close association between the mechanisms which, when damaged, result in slowness of movement and slowness of thought, and that these are to be found in the medial basal areas of the cerebral hemispheres which, in closed head injury, are especially vulnerable both to shear strain damage and to secondary infarction.

7 Cranial Nerve Injuries, Vertigo and Headache

The frequency with which persistent signs of cranial nerve injury were found amongst the consecutive series of patients is recorded in table 7.1. The main concern of this study has been the assessment of disability. In considering evidence of residual cranial nerve damage it seemed justifiable, therefore, to record differing degrees of impaired function of each nerve appropriate to the disability caused. A minor degree of impairment of the sense of smell was not only difficult to relate with certainty to the injury but also of negligible inconvenience compared with minor degrees of double vision due to residual external ocular muscle weakness. For these reasons only complete loss of the sense of smell, that is for gas, faeces and onions or, when tested, for asafoetida, and then only if the patient was certain that this had been present since the injury, was reckoned as 'disability' due to injury of the first cranial nerves. Similar considerations applied to the assessment of deafness. Only in cases where there was total or near total hearing loss on one side which had persisted since the accident has hearing loss been discussed. Disability due to traumatic vestibular dysfunction has been studied separately. Residual signs of other cranial nerve lesions have been recorded even when these were minimal.

Anosmia

The highest prevalence of permanent traumatic anosmia was found amongst patients who were older than twenty-five years at the time of their injury. Although not shown in table 7.1, this trend was also apparent in injuries sustained over the age of forty. There was no constant relationship to the severity of the injury assessed by the duration of post-traumatic amnesia, nor, apparently, to the side of head impact or skull fracture, although it may be that significant differences were obscured by the small number of patients available for analysis within each age group. There was an overall prevalence of persistent anosmia of 20 per cent amongst those whose injuries had been complicated by surface compression or brain penetration, compared with a 12 per cent prevalence amongst those whose injuries had been uncomplicated.

The attempt to examine the relationship between anosmia recorded in the hospital notes during convalescence and at re-examination 10 or more years later was abandoned when it became clear that, especially amongst the more severely injured, there had been an underestimate of transient loss of smell and taste. Complete loss, which had gone unrecorded at the time of discharge from hospital, was frequently found at re-examination. Where

Table 7.1 Prevalence of persisting cranial nerve lesions

Cranial nerve	Age at injury 5–15 (9)* (39)†		Age at injury 16–45 (50)* (143)†		Age at injury 46+ (18)* (32)†	
	Complicated	Uncomplicated	Complicated	Uncomplicated	Complicated	Uncomplicated
I 20%* 12%†						
PTA (weeks)						
<4	(8)	2(32)	3(30)10%	7(115) 6%	5(11) 46%	10(22)45%
>4	1(1)	(7)	4(20)20%	3(28)11%	2(7) 28%	2(10)20%
Head impact‡						
Frontal	1(3)	(11)	4(19)22%	4(76) 5%	(3)	3(13)23%
Lateral	(2)	(8)	(15)	1(13) 8%	2(2)100%	1(3)33%
Occipital/parietal	(4)	1(12)	2(16)12%	4(38)10%	5(13) 38%	8(15)54%
Skull fracture						
Yes	1(8)	1(25)	4(45) 9%	7(75) 9%	7(13) 54%	10(25)38%
No	(1)	1(14)	3(5)60%	(68)	(5)	2(7)25%
II 3%* 3%†						
PTA (weeks)						
<4				1 bilateral field defect 1 N36 field defect 3 blind one eye		
>4			2 blind one eye	1 N24 field defect		
Head impact						
Frontal			1 blind one eye	1 blind one eye 1 N36 field defect		
Lateral			1 blind one eye	1 N24 field defect		
Occipital/parietal				1 blind one eye		
Skull fracture						
Yes			2 blind one eye	2 blind one eye 2 N26/24 field defects 1 blind one eye 1 N36 bilat field defects		
No						

Table 7.1 — continued

Cranial nerve	Age at injury 5–15 (9)* (39)†		Age at injury 16–45 (50)* (143)†		Age at injury 46+ (18)* (32)†	
	Complicated	Uncomplicated	Complicated	Uncomplicated	Complicated	Uncomplicated
III 8%* 6%†						
PTA (weeks)						
<4				8		3
>4			4	2	2	
Head impact						
Frontal			1	5		2
Lateral			3	2		
Occipital/parietal				3	2	1
Skull fracture						
Yes			3	7	1	2
No			1	1	1	1
VI 5%* 2%†						
PTA (weeks)						
<4			3	3		1
>4			1			
Head impact						
Frontal			3	1		1
Lateral				1		
Occipital/parietal			1	1		
Skull fracture						
Yes				2		
No				1		1

Table 7.1 continued overleaf

Table 7.1 — continued

	Age at injury 5–15 (9)* (39)†		Age at injury 16–45 (50)* (143)†		Age at injury 46+ (18)* (32)†	
	Complicated	Uncomplicated	Complicated	Uncomplicated	Complicated	Uncomplicated
VII 3%* 3%†						
PTA (weeks)						
<4			1	5		
>4			1	2		
Head impact						
Frontal			1	1		
Lateral				3		
Occipital/parietal				3		
Skull fracture						
Yes			1			
No				7		

Consecutive series total 291; complicated injuries 77; uncomplicated injuries 214.
* Numbers so marked indicate complicated injuries.
† Numbers so marked indicate uncomplicated injuries.
‡ Discrepancy in numbers due to uncertainty about site of impact in a few cases.

anosmia had been recorded in the notes but was not present later, patients were asked to describe their recollection of this impaired perception of smell and taste and how long it took to recover.

Recollection was uncertain in many cases, and for this reason no overall assessments were possible. From the information provided by those who did remember it was clear, however, that the majority had recovered within 6 months. A number of patients, after having experienced longer periods of hyposmia recovered a serviceable, although slightly impaired, perception of smell and taste over the course of as many as 2–3 years. There was no patient in either the consecutive or selected series who had died from coal gas poisoning as a result of anosmia, although one elderly demented patient did survive such an accident.

Optic Nerves and Chiasm

The overall prevalence of persisting field defects with impaired visual acuity or blindness was 3 per cent in both complicated and uncomplicated injuries. As with the first cranial nerve, age appeared to be a significant determinant since all had been injured between the ages of sixteen and forty-five years. Numbers were too small to assess the relevance of the severity of the injury, side of head impact, and presence or absence of skull fracture. Complete blindness of one eye persisted in five patients, and in each the optic disc was atrophic. There was some attenuation of the retinal vessels, but in no case was there evidence of retinal artery or branch occlusion. There were two patients with bilateral field defects, optic atrophy and reduced visual acuity. In the first there was complete loss of the upper fields and lower temporal quadrants in both eyes and visual acuity in either eye was reduced to reading N34 print. The other patient had lost the lower half field and peripheral temporal sector of one eye, together with a similar peripheral sector of the homonymous field of the other eye. Visual acuity was reduced only to N14 in the worst eye and was normal in the best. The first case had no demonstrable fracture of the skull and in the second there were frontal fractures. In addition there were seven patients in the same age group when injured, with optic atrophy but normal visual acuity, and no field defect on confrontation with a 5-mm white pin, who had been recorded as having some impairment of visual acuity during convalescence. There were two similar patients in the oldest age group. There was only one patient blinded by traumatic retinal detachment whilst another had his visual acuity severely impaired by commotio retinae, although this later resolved completely.

Varying degrees of optic atrophy, usually in both eyes, was a common finding amongst patients still decerebrate or severely disabled by athetoid pseudobulbar lesions. Where there was adequate cooperation for testing to be carried out in these cases, none had unilateral field defects. In most of them the degree of dementia prevented any assessment of visual acuity, and field defects to menace were usually on the side of the more severely paralysed limbs. The majority of these patients were from the selected series who had suffered prolonged unconsciousness, and are not included in table 7.1, which deals with the prevalence of these persisting cranial nerve lesions.

One patient with a chiasmal lesion complained of increasing difficulty in seeing since the injury. Apparently he was eventually unable to read large print, although he had been able to do so for some weeks after the injury, and he finally professed himself to be totally blind. His brother, however, commented on the discrepant fact that he was able to find his way about without difficulty. This was the only case seen in which the question arose of progressive traumatic optic neuritis attributable to the basal arachnoiditis mentioned by Walsh and Hoyt (1969).

In addition, there were a number of patients whose visual acuity tested with reading type, even wearing their own spectacles, was worse than N8 in one or the other eye. Improvement in acuity, using a pinhole, was often demonstrable, but without more sophisticated techniques of assessment of visual function it was not possible to assess the relevance of the head injury, and it does not seem likely that considering these further will serve any useful purpose.

Ocular Palsies

There was a marginal difference in the frequency with which persisting evidence of third nerve palsies was found in complicated and uncomplicated injuries. The prevalence was 8 per cent in the former and 6 per cent in the latter. Residual lateral rectus weakness was similarly slightly commoner amongst those with complicated injuries, the respective prevalences being 5 per cent for complicated and 2 per cent for uncomplicated injury. The same relative importance of age in determining persisting external ocular palsies is seen. Diplopia was only a minor inconvenience in most cases and apparent only on gaze in one direction; surgical treatment had only been resorted to in four patients. It was surprising how few complained of their double vision when asked to describe persisting disabilities. The fact that there was more evidence of third nerve damage than sixth presumably reflects the fact that the latter was more frequently a false localising sign due to raised intracranial pressure causing no permanent injury to the nerve. The oculomotor nerve appears not only more vulnerable to permanent damage from raised intracranial pressure, but also to be injured more frequently as a direct result of skull fracture. There were only two certain cases of superior oblique palsies found at the time of re-examination, and these were both associated with residual partial third nerve palsies. In three patients residual muscle weakness was associated with orbital fractures and intra-orbital haematomas. Despite what had clearly been severe damage to the orbit, the lasting disability due to diplopia was minimal in each.

It is likely that all the third and sixth nerve palsies developing during the acute stage after injury were recorded in the notes. Unfortunately, it cannot be assumed that all had been abstracted from the case records and no attempt will be made to compare the overall incidence with persisting signs. It was, however, clear that in the majority of cases where there had been third and sixth nerve palsies recorded at the time of injury and none was found at re-examination, recovery had taken place within a few months, often while the patient was still in hospital, and invariably within 6 months.

An interesting observation, but again impossible to quantify because of the uncertain proportion recorded, and also because of possible selective abstraction of data, was the frequent occurrence at the time of injury of disconjugate and other abnormal eye movements. These, together with inequality of pupils not associated with third or sixth nerve palsies, suggested internuclear and supranuclear involvement in the brainstem. There were three cases of impaired conjugate ocular movement, suggesting internuclear ophthalmoplegia, still demonstrable 10 years after injury.

Trigeminal Nerve

A long-standing sensory deficit due to injury of this nerve was a rarity. There was no case in which all three divisions of the nerve were permanently damaged. In three cases the infra-orbital branch was involved and in two of these there were associated maxillary fractures. In the other case there had been an anterior skull fracture. There were two patients whose sensory loss was in the distribution of the supra-orbital nerve. Tarsorrhaphies had been necessary for combined facial paralysis and trigeminal sensory loss in two patients. Both of these had recovered sensibility, although there had been no similar recovery of the facial palsies. There was no case of post-traumatic trigeminal neuralgia or causalgia.

Facial Nerve

The prevalence of residual facial nerve palsies of any degree has been recorded both because it was a simple assessment to make clinically and also because, even when slight, it constituted a serious cosmetic disability; in both complicated and uncomplicated injuries it was 3 per cent. The relationship to age is as striking as for other cranial nerve palsies. There were only two patients with persisting complete facial palsies, and another five who had a degree of aberrant re-innervation and weakness which could be considered a severe cosmetic disability. There was one patient with gustatory hyperhidrosis and two with crocodile tears. Most of these facial palsies were associated with parietal or lateral fractures of the skull, and there was no case of persisting facial palsy where the skull had not been fractured.

Hearing

Total or near total loss of hearing on one side had persisted since injury in only three cases. Two were associated with fractures running into the petrous bone and one with a frontal fracture. Mild degrees of impairment of hearing in one or both ears, and dating from the injury, were common complaints. These were confirmed by routine clinical tests and in the majority of cases appeared to be conductive in type. A number of these patients had chronic otitis media which antedated the head injury. In many patients over the age of forty-six at the time of injury there was no certain means of deciding whether the mild defects of hearing they attributed to the head injury were not due rather to normal ageing. Therefore, apart from noting that total permanent loss of hearing was extremely rare and minor degrees of impaired hearing very common after severe closed head injury, on the evidence collected here no more detailed statement than this can be made about traumatic auditory lesions.

Lower Cranial Nerve Palsies

There were only two patients recorded as sustaining cranial nerve palsies involving the ninth, tenth, eleventh and twelfth nerves. In one case all four nerves on one side were paralysed. A basal fracture had extended into the foramen magnum. There were no signs of these palsies when the patient was re-examined 12 years later. One other patient with paralysis of the sterno-mastoid muscle on one side, recorded at the time of injury, was found to have slight atrophy of this same muscle when re-examined 15 years later, but no disability as a result.

Vertigo

This almost invariably took the form of transient, but often violent, sensations of rotation, and less commonly swaying movements causing momentary imbalance provoked by movement. Almost without exception the symptom was provoked by looking upwards, but rising from a chair, turning quickly to either side, and, rarely, turning over in bed, were also liable to induce transient vertigo. Positional tests were not used to confirm the vertigo, nor was it considered justifiable to subject these patients to standard tests of vestibular function. This, and the fact that vertigo was both incompletely recorded in the hospital notes and selectively abstracted for this study, especially when more severe neural disabilities overshadowed this relatively minor symptom, reduces the accuracy of the incidence of transient vertigo noted here. There were only two patients with persisting positional vertigo severe enough to make their occupation hazardous. They were both painters and decorators. One had continued at his work despite his disability, whilst the other had changed his job.

Vertigo which lasted only weeks or months, compared with vertigo which still persisted at the time of re-examination, is related to age in table 7.2.

Table 7.2   Positional vertigo, age at injury and type of injury

| | Age at injury | | | |
	5–15	16–45	46+	Totals
Uncomplicated injury				
Total number of patients	39	143	32	214
Number with vertigo				
lasting weeks or months	3	20	7	30
Number with vertigo				
persisting 10 years or more	5	42	9	56 (26%)
Complicated injury				
Total number of patients	9	50	18	77
Number with vertigo				
lasting weeks or months	0	8	4	12
Number with vertigo				
persisting 10 years or more	4	9	2	15 (19%)
Complicated and uncomplicated injury				
Total number of patients	48	193	50	291
Number with vertigo				
persisting 10 years or more	9	51	11	71
Percentage	19%	26%	22%	24%

Nearly one-quarter of the patients were still experiencing positional vertigo more than 10 years after injury. It can be seen that a head injury complicated by surface compression or brain penetration does not increase the likelihood of persisting positional vertigo, and age seems irrelevant. Most patients still suffering from this symptom had been conditioned by experience to move sufficiently circumspectly so as to be seldom troubled by it. In table 7.3 the severity of the injury, judged by length of post-traumatic amnesia, is ex-

Table 7.3   Persisting positional vertigo and severity of injury

| | Duration PTA | |
	Less than 3 weeks	3 weeks and longer
Total number of patients	150	141
Number with vertigo		
persisting 10 years or more	32	39
Percentage	22%	28%

amined as a factor determining the persistence of vertigo. There is no indication that a more severe injury is more likely to result in prolonged positional vertigo amongst patients whose injury was already severe enough to cause traumatic amnesia lasting for a week.

Headache

The incidence of post-traumatic headache in this study is likely to be an underestimate, as in the case of vertigo and some of the cranial nerve lesions, and for the same reasons. This again is due partly to the fact that the more severe the injury the less frequently was headache recorded in the notes, and the less often was the patient able to recall that he had suffered from headaches when asked about it at interview. In general no association with age could be discerned, nor with surface brain compression or brain penetration complicating the injury. On the other hand, a striking finding was that persistence of headache related closely to its character and severity. Table 7.4

Table 7.4   Persistence of post-traumatic headache and age at injury

Type of headache	Persistence	
	Less than 2 years	Several years
Number of patients with		
Classical migraine: hemicranial, with or without visual aura, prostrating, nauseating and with photophobia	0	8 (2 further cases of post-traumatic migrainous neuralgia)
'Migrainous vascular': severe, throbbing, generalised, more or less prostrating	3	18
Severe non-throbbing, localised or generalised, non-prostrating	19	22
Minor headaches	36	10

distinguishes between four different types of headache and shows their relation to its duration. It appears that the more severe the headache, the more likely it is to last for longer than a year, and conversely, that the less severe the headache the more likely it is to clear up within months of the injury.

The relationships between the severity of the injury, judged by the duration of post-traumatic amnesia, and the type of headache and its persistence, are examined in table 7.5. Although there is some suggestion that with increasing severity of injury there is a greater chance of severe headaches persisting, this

Table 7.5 Severity and persistence of post-traumatic headache and severity and type of injury

	Classical migraine or prostrating 'vascular'		Severe non-throbbing non-prostrating		Minor headaches	
	<2 year	2 year +	<2 year	2 year +	<2 year	2 year +
Uncomplicated injury Number of patients with PTA						
<2 weeks	2	7	9	3	11	5
2 weeks +	1	12	7	11	13	1
Complicated injury Number of patients with PTA						
<2 weeks	0	5	2	2	2	1
2 weeks +	0	2	1	6	10	3
Uncomplicated and complicated injury Number of patients with PTA						
<2 weeks	2	12	11	5	13	6
2 weeks +	1	14	8	17	23	4

	Classical migraine or prostrating 'vascular' or severe non-throbbing, non-prostrating		Minor headaches	
	<2 year	2 year +	<2 year	2 year +
Uncomplicated and complicated injury Number of patients with PTA				
<2 weeks	13	17	13	6
2 weeks +	9	31	23	4

is not always so. More severe, long-lasting headaches are found among those who have longer post-traumatic amnesias, but the least severe and shortest-lasting type of headache also occurs in patients who had longer post-traumatic amnesias.

It appears that classical migraine, that is, violent prostrating headaches, with or without aura, but associated in most cases with nausea and photophobia, may cease after severe head injury, increase in frequency for a period of 2 years or so, or develop for the first time. Vascular headaches which were severe and more or less prostrating, and which, characteristically, throbbed, and might be described as migraine variants, were longer lasting in general than in minor headaches. Some anecdotal data were of interest. There were seven patients who lost for good the non-specific headaches they had experienced for many years before injury. One lost her classical migraine, another lost her morning tension headaches for a period of several weeks. These last two patients both had a mild frontal personality change, the first permanent and the second temporary. One patient had fewer tension headaches after the head injury than she had had for years before. Several patients had experienced recurrent severe headaches, apparently provoked by tension, only since the injury. It was difficult to be certain that the character of these headaches differed from those they had experienced before.

A number of the more severely injured patients stated firmly that they had never known what a headache was after their injury. This was a statement also made by several patients who, judging by the length of their post-traumatic amnesia, had been the least severely concussed.

Discussion

The infrequency with which evidence of cranial nerve lesions persists long after severe closed head injury has been alluded to briefly by several of the authors whose papers were reviewed in an earlier chapter, and the observations made in this study are in general agreement. None of these authors, however, commented on an increased prevalence of anosmia with increasing age at the time of injury. The relative tendency for children to be spared optic nerve injury and to make excellent recovery from ocular palsies has been noted by Hooper (1951) and the generally good prognosis for ocular palsies was commented on by Hughes (1964). Mealey (1968) found that facial palsies were relatively uncommon after closed head injuries in childhood.

It is perhaps surprising that the prevalence of optic nerve and chiasmal injury is so little higher amongst these patients with very severe injuries than Turner (1943) found. In a series of 1000 cases of all grades of severity of 'indirect' optic nerve injury he found only 25 cases, that is, a prevalence only marginally less than in the present study. Recovery of function in the long-term cannot be the explanation.

It has been shown experimentally by Hirakawa, Hashizume, Nakamura and Sano (1971) that even minor impact forces may momentarily cause depression of the roof of the optic canal, and presumably damage optic nerves and their vasculature. It may be that the ischaemic infarcts found by Crompton (1970) in a high proportion of optic nerves and chiasms in patients dying of their injuries were caused by shear strain acceleration forces which are seldom survived. The negligibly greater frequency with which certain evidence of optic nerve or chiasmal lesions was found in the most severely brain-damaged patients in the selected series of cases studied here suggests that this is so and, moreover, provides further support for the view that secondary infarction rather than primary trauma is more often the cause of severe neural disability after closed head injury.

In a study of the site of the lesion responsible for hearing loss after blunt head injury Lehnhardt (1974) followed a series of 20 patients over a 4-year period. He noted that improvement did not occur with time. In his view the evidence he put forward favoured lesions in the brainstem as an explanation of the neural component of the post-traumatic deafness in his cases. Tests of vestibular function carried out by Toglia, Rosenberg and Ronis (1970) in a series of 568 patients who had sustained closed head injuries of varying degrees of severity, showed that, although patients might lose their vertiginous symptoms at any time from months to years after injury, the disturbances of vestibular function remained permanently demonstrable by appropriate techniques.

In a study of 78 patients 2–17 years after severe closed head injury, Szmeja, Pruszewicz, Tokarz, Zwozdzia and Obrebowski (1974) were similarly able to show that the characteristics of the auditory and vestibular dysfunction were little different either shortly or many years after injury, indicating that the damage was irrecoverable, although the patients could adjust to it. In a review of the aetiology of positional vertigo Harrison and Ozsohinoglu (1972) have also pointed out the persistent nature of much traumatic positional vertigo, and although they felt it more likely to be permanent in older patients, as was not found in this present study, none of these authors comment on the degree of disability that symptoms ultimately cause, but all note the distressing character of movement-induced vertigo in the short-term.

The characteristics of late traumatic headache have been reviewed by Wolff (1963) and, more recently, by Nick and Sicard-Nick (1965). These authors draw attention to the incidence of migrainous types, which the former found in 7 per cent of the cases they reviewed and the latter in 25 per cent. Tubbs and Potter (1970) reported an increasing incidence of early post-traumatic headache with severity of injury in a series of patients suffering from relatively trivial injury, judged by the standards of the present study. None of these authors comment on the long-term prognosis for the various forms of headache which follow trauma to the head.

8 Pituitary and Hypothalamic Disorders

It has been well established in recent years that traumatic haemorrhage and infarction in the supra-optic region of the hypothalamus are almost invariable findings in patients who have died as a result and within a few days of their head injuries and they are commonly seen also in the adjacent infundibular region. The extent to which these lesions, or rather lesser damage in the same areas, is likely to result in disordered pituitary and hypothalamic function in the long-term amongst those who survive does not appear to have been studied systematically before. It is clear, however, that in those who survive severe head injury, damage to the hypothalamus must have been relatively common judged by the frequency with which hyperphagia and polyuria occur. Less certainly, the post-traumatic electrolyte imbalances, particularly of sodium and chloride ions, may be due to impaired production of the peptide releasers of corticotrophin from supra-optic and paraventricular nuclei. The occasional case of acute and otherwise unexplained hypotension within days of the injury, which appears to respond to treatment with hydrocortisone also raises the possibility of impaired hypothalamo-hypophyseal function.

In this study an attempt was made to assess evidence of persisting endocrine disorder both by systematic recording of clinically observable signs of hypopituitarism, obesity and abnormalities of stature, and also by questioning patients and their relatives as to sexual function before and after injury, abnormalities of micturition, and indications of sub-fertility. So far as sexual performance was concerned the original intention to question each patient and the spouse in detail was abandoned when it seemed, particularly in the more severely disabled, that such enquiry might appear little more than misplaced impertinence. In rather more than half the cases, when it was judged that no distress would be caused, these questions were asked, so that there is information available for this selected portion of the series, most of them the less severely damaged. With this exception the facts relating to long-lasting evidence of pituitary and hypothalamic function are available for both the consecutive and the selected series of patients.

The same cannot be said of the incidence of disordered anterior and posterior pituitary function during the acute and convalescent stages after the injury. It is more than likely that minor degrees of increased urinary output and increased appetite were not recorded in the hospital notes. Also, since the principal concern in abstracting data from these records was to provide a detailed description of the evolution and progress of the neurological state of the patients, it may well be, again more often in severely injured patients, that a number of comments referring to this evidence of hypothalamic disorder were overlooked. No attempt was made to abstract data referring to electrolyte imbalance.

Hypothalamic and Adenohypophyseal Functions

At the time of re-examination there was only one patient with a certain diagnosis of *anterior hypopituitarism*. This was a boy of ten who had been receiving supplementary cortisone acetate since the diagnosis of anterior hypopituitarism had been confirmed by appropriate investigations a year after his head injury. At that time he was still obese and drinking large quantities of fluid indicating also a persisting disorder of neurohypophyseal function and bilateral damage to the satiety centres in the floor of the rostral hypothalamus.

Another man of thirty-four, when examined 12 years after his injury, was found to have a smooth skin, relative beardlessness and scanty body hair, together with the pallid obesity suggestive of hypopituitarism. Within the past year a fit had resulted in another head injury complicated by a subdural haematoma. This had been effectively evacuated; then, after a delay of some weeks, his condition had progressively deteriorated. It seemed likely that this was due to a communicating hydrocephalus, but further investigation was not undertaken by the neurosurgeon to whom he was sent and the doubtful clinical diagnosis was not confirmed.

In addition to these two patients there were four men and one woman whose appearance suggested uncertainly that there might have been some disorder of anterior pituitary function. The men were smaller and less well bearded than normal for their ages, and in two cases this was in obvious contrast to the appearance of the father. The adolescent woman was considerably smaller and plumper than her mother or her father but her endocrine system was otherwise evidently normal in that she had already required two therapeutic abortions for illegitimate pregnancies, a sequel to severe frontal personality damage. All had been injured before the age of fifteen.

Minor degrees of hypothalamic-pituitary hypofunction were sought by examining the prevalence of childlessness amongst married women of child-bearing age, loss of libido and potency in men, and the number of single men who might reasonably have been expected to have married and were not obviously mentally or physically at such a disadvantage as a result of their injuries as to limit their chances of marriage. Six women were childless despite attempts to conceive for more than 10 years. Confirmatory evidence that this was due to their own infertility rather than the husbands' was available in only three cases. None had been severely injured and in only two had evidence of hypothalamic injury been abstracted from the case notes. In both these patients the evidence consisted of transient hyperphagia and in one case there had been transient polyuria as well.

The significance of the loss of libido and potency is difficult to assess in relation to pituitary hypofunction where this is not otherwise overt. In addition, where sexual function was lost it was difficult to distinguish between loss of libido and loss of potency. In this selective enquiry the only fact that emerged was that, amongst those who were questioned, age at the time of injury appeared to be the most important factor determining permanent post-traumatic loss of sexual function. There were three patients injured between the ages of twenty-six and thirty-five who remained impotent thereafter, 14 injured between the ages of thirty-six and forty-five, and five who were older than this when they were injured who never recovered sexual function. In none of these cases was there any record of diabetes insipidus or hyperphagia following injury and only six of them were still seriously disabled as a result of their neural lesions. In interesting contrast there were 13 patients who had experienced a temporary or permanent increase in libido and sexual performance after their injuries. Most of these had a persisting impairment of day-to-day memory of a relatively minor degree, and in three there was an associated mild frontal personality change.

There were six men of marriageable age injured between the ages of five and fifteen who were still single more than 10 years later, 12 injured between the ages of sixteen and twenty-five who were still single, and nine injured between the ages of twenty-six and thirty-five, of whom five had been single for over 10 years at a time when they might reasonably have been expected to have been married even before injury. Of these 27 patients two had been recorded as having transient hyperphagia when recovering from their injuries and one diabetes insipidus.

In addition there were two other patients who had been diagnosed as suffering from acute pituitary failure shortly after injury when they became inexplicably hypotensive. These had both received steroids for a short period and had made complete recoveries. There was no evidence of hypopituitarism clinically in either case. Indeed one of them had clearly more than adequate libido as evidenced by repeated convictions for indecent exposure, this being one manifestation of his severe frontal personality change.

Hypothalamic and Neurohypophyseal Functions

A diagnosis of *diabetes insipidus* made on the basis of polyuria with or without urinary or serum confirmation was noted in eight cases out of the 291 re-examined patients in the consecutive series. The incidence is set out in table 8.1.

Table 8.1 Incidence of hyperphagia and diabetes insipidus after closed head injury

	Age at injury	
	5–25 years	26–55 years
Number with hyperphagia	13	3
Total number	149	142
Percentage	9%	2%
Number with diabetes insipidus	5	3
Percentage	3.5%	2%

Consecutive series, 291 patients.

The relationship of this manifestation of neurohypophyseal damage to age, the severity of the injury as judged by the duration of post-traumatic amnesia and of decerebration, and to the evidence of persisting memory impairment, personality change and physical disability due to neural lesions in both the consecutive and the selected series is set out in tables 8.2 and 8.3.

Table 8.2 Hypothalamic hyperphagia and diabetes insipidus after closed head injury in relation to age and severity of injury

	Age at injury	
Consecutive series, 291 patients	5–25 years	26–55 years
Number with hyperphagia	13	3
Total number	149	142
Percentage	9%	2%
Number with diabetes insipidus	5	3
Percentage	3.5%	2%

	PTA	
Consecutive and selected series, 331 patients	<4 weeks	>4 weeks
Number with hyperphagia	4	18
Total number	22	
Percentage	18%	82%
Number with diabetes insipidus	5	4
Total number	9	
Percentage	55%	45%

	Coma	
	<3 weeks	>3 weeks
Number with hyperphagia	6	16
Percentage	27%	73%
Number with diabetes insipidus	6	3
Percentage	65%	35%

	Decerebration	
	No	Yes
Number with hyperphagia	9	13
Percentage	40%	60%
Number with diabetes insipidus	5	4
Percentage	55%	45%

	Deterioration after admission	
	No	Yes
Number with hyperphagia	17	5
Percentage	77%	23%
Number with diabetes insipidus	4	5
Percentage	44%	56%

Table 8.3 Hypothalamic hyperphagia and diabetes insipidus after injury in relation to persisting memory impairment and personality disorder and to the pattern of persisting central neural lesions in both series of patients

	Pattern of mental disorder				
	Frontal, irritable and forgetful	Frontal and/or irritable	Frontal, or irritable and forgetful	Forgetful only	None
Hyperphagia	9	3	4	4	1
Diabetes insipidus	4	1	1	2	1

	Pattern of neural lesions				
	Decerebrate	Athetoid pseudobulbar	Brainstem cerebellar	Hemiparetic	None
Hyperphagia	0	4	10 (all severe)	6 (5 minimal)	2
Diabetes insipidus	0	1	5 (3 severe)	2 (minimal)	1

It would appear that whatever measure of severity of injury is taken, there are more patients who develop transient diabetes insipidus amongst those who have been severely injured and amongst those who were in the younger age groups at the time of injury. It seems likely that these observations are closely related in that survival after severe acceleration injury becomes less common with increasing age.

In four of these patients the polyuria occurred in the second week after injury and in three cases in the third to eighth week. In one patient it developed within a week of injury, whilst in another it was confirmed, together with both clinical and biochemical evidence of anterior pituitary hypofunction, only $1\frac{1}{2}$ years after injury. In only two cases was it necessary to treat the patients with pitressin. One of these was the patient already referred to with panhypopituitarism. The other sustained a comminuted depressed right frontal skull fracture extending into the orbit and sinuses, together with fractures of the right malar bone and both mandibles. He developed a right-sided pulsating proptosis suggesting a carotico-cavernous shunt which subsided spontaneously. His severe diabetes insipidus declared itself in the third week and required parenteral therapy with pitressin tannate. He underwent a craniotomy and dural repair at 6 weeks. His convalescence thereafter was complicated only by continuing polyuria requiring regular pitressin injections after his discharge from hospital. Two months after the injury he decided to visit some relatives and failed to attend his general practitioner for further injections. He described his experience for about 10 days thereafter as 'torture'. His excruciating thirst subsequently ceased as did his polyuria, and although since then he had regularly had to get out of bed once a night to micturate, as he had not done before his injury, there were no other symptoms to suggest diabetes insipidus. None of the other patients had symptoms which were certainly attributable to neurohypophyseal hypofunction within a few weeks of injury, though most continued to need to micturate at night and experienced diurnal frequency for several months.

It is difficult to determine the extent to which minor degrees of impaired neurohypophyseal function were the cause of nocturnal incontinence, nocturia which had not been present before, and distressing diurnal frequency which lasted for several months or years. This is particularly so because of the available evidence, both experimental in mammals and clinical and pathological in man, that both frontal and septal areas are involved in the integration of the act of micturition in addition to the rostral hypothalamus. This subject has been reviewed by Andrew and Nathan (1965). They draw attention to cases in which tumours and standard leucotomies have damaged white matter between the superior frontal and anterior cingulate gyri, and to tumours of the septal region associated with urgency and frequency of micturition. Actual incontinence of urine and faeces, usually without awareness, may occur with more severe damage, but it causes embarrassment and distress indicating that it is not simply due to frontal anergia and apathy.

With the exception of the frontal convexities these are the areas invariably damaged by both primary trauma and secondary infarction in severe head injuries. There were patients seen in the present study whose urinary incontinence occurred without bladder sensation. This, in the presence of full consciousness and without severe dementia, usually lasted several months after the injury and, on the above evidence, seems more likely to be due to damage in the frontal white matter than in the neurohypophysis. Approximately one-fifth of those who were injured before they were fifteen were enuretic for months, and a few for years, after their injury. Amongst those over the age of sixteen at the time of injury about one-tenth suffered in this way. There was no clear description in any of these cases of typical incontinence without awareness. In the older patients impairment of sexual function was commonly associated.

Nocturia and diurnal frequency without incontinence occurred in a small proportion of cases within each age group and although in most these symptoms ceased within the first year, in a small number they persisted indefinitely. The majority of those with urinary symptoms which lasted either several months or persisted indefinitely had evidence of persisting day-to-day memory defects, frontal personality change or continuing and uncharacteristic irritability. Of passing interest were five patients with pre-traumatic enuresis cured by the injury. In one this was certainly due to the training he had received in hospital, but it was unexplained in the others. On re-examination none of these patients was disabled either by neural lesions or by mental changes.

Hyperphagia was noted in the case records of 16 patients in the consecutive series and of six in the selected series whose coma had been prolonged for a month or more. The incidence of this symptom in the consecutive series is noted in table 8.1. The relationship to age and to the severity of injury in both series of patients is set out in tables 8.2 and 8.3. As in the case of diabetes insipidus, but seen more clearly with the larger numbers, it is apparent that the younger the patient and the more severe the injury, the more likely it is that hypothalamic hyperphagia will occur. The most probable explanation is that, similarly, only the young survive with any frequency injuries severe enough to cause these lesions.

The fact that the optic nerves, chiasm and tract are anatomically so closely related to the hypothalamic region suggests that injuries to one structure might occur when the other is damaged.

There were two patients who had had hyperphagia who also both had optic nerve lesions, severe athetoid pseudobulbar syndromes, profound personality change and intellectual impairment, together with optic atrophy and field defects in one or both eyes, that were clearly due neither to retinal nor cerebral damage. Another grossly obese patient with severe optic atrophy on both sides was so profoundly demented and uncooperative that it was impossible to confirm what seemed likely to be field defects in both eyes which were not explicable on the basis of hemisphere damage. One patient who had had transient post-traumatic diabetes insipidus was left with a unilateral field defect and atrophy of the optic disc of that eye.

Discussion

In a review of traumatic hypothalamic and pituitary pathology and an assessment of the frequency with which it occurred Treip (1970) drew attention to the incidence of haemorrhages of varying sizes, but mostly petechial, found in the region of the supra-optic nucleus and less commonly elsewhere in the hypothalamus. At the same time he noted the infrequency with which anterior hypopituitarism due to trauma had been confirmed histologically in those surviving the immediate effects of their head injury. This, he concluded, was good evidence that infarction of the pars distalis sufficient to cause hypopituitarism was seldom survived for any length of time, possibly because of the severity of the associated injuries. On the other hand, he felt that lesser degrees of hypothalamic damage might be less immediately fatal and allow deficiency syndromes to develop later on. According to Okuma, Oda and Matushita (1973), who reviewed previous reports up to that date, there had only been 20 adequately documented cases of *anterior pituitary insufficiency* after head injury. They described another case of a man who developed the first symptoms of his anterior hypopituitarism 2 months after injury and who remained undiagnosed for another 6 years. This delay in onset and slow development thereafter seems characteristic of post-traumatic anterior pituitary failure and has been further documented by, amongst others, Bevilacqua and Fornaciari (1975), Wolfe and Schalch (1973) and Majumdar and Bhushan (1975). It is difficult to see what relationship there was between the very minor head injury sustained by the patient and the 'traumatic' panhypopituitarism reported by Goldman and Jacobs (1960). The one certain case described in the present study was typically delayed in onset until the second year. In a second case the diagnosis was suggested on clinical grounds alone when the patient was re-examined for the purpose of this study 12 years after injury. His condition then was so parlous due to the effects of a second head injury that no further investigations were undertaken by the neurosurgeon whose opinion had been sought, and no confirmation of the possible diagnosis is available. Other clinical evidence for impaired anterior pituitary function sought in the present study included unusually small stature (among those injured in childhood), deficient secondary sexual characteristics, impotence, failure to marry and sterility. These were infrequently encountered and did not seem likely to be outside the number encountered in routine clinical practice. It may be reasonable therefore to conclude that injuries likely to result in the development of late anterior hypopituitarism due to head injury are remarkably rare. It is not the author's impression that any patient in the present series died as a result of acute pituitary failure at the time of injury.

Similarly, traumatic *diabetes insipidus* was noted in the case records of only eight patients in the consecutive series in the present study. This incidence is comparable with that noted by others. In reviewing 5000 cases of closed head injury Porter and Miller (1948) found 13 cases of diabetes insipidus and added five more cases. Of these 18 cases, 13 had post-traumatic amnesia lasting longer than a week, indicating the severity of the injury required to impair significantly neurohypophyseal function, and no doubt explaining the rather higher incidence in the present series of patients. In their review of the condition Orthner and Meyer (1967) concluded that although minor degrees of polyuria due to diabetes insipidus might be overlooked, it occurred only after severe head injury. They reported an incidence of 1 in 200. Symptoms persisting longer than a few weeks were present in only one case in the present series and this patient also had anterior pituitary hypofunction. Although in one case pitressin was needed for a few weeks after discharge from hospital, the condition in the remaining patients was self-limiting. There were no other longer-lasting cases.

The same may be said of *hypothalamic hyperphagia*, and the frequency of this condition would appear to be no greater judging by the review of the literature by Wowern (1966). In this study there were only four cases in the consecutive series who remained obese after their head injury but had not been so before. In all the other patients noted to be eating excessively and to be putting on inordinate amounts of weight after their injuries, this ceased within a year or two. Two of the patients who remained obese were profoundly demented with severe 'frontal' apathy.

It- is virtually certain that post-traumatic hyperphagia is attributable to injury on both sides of the hypothalamus, involving the paired satiety centres first proposed by Hetherington and Ranson (1940). An exceptionally well-documented case of post-traumatic hypothalamic obesity reported by Miyasaki, Miyachi, Arimitzu, Kita and Yoshida (1972) confirmed the situation of the secondary hypothalamic infarcts at post-mortem. These involved the paraventricular area on both sides, which are the sites of the satiety centres. The region lateral to this was also infarcted on one side but the same region on the other side and the appetite centre there was spared. The woman had sustained a very severe injury, had deteriorated in conscious level and responsiveness for some days, and had then lived for 2 years, being grossly obese and eating voraciously until her death in cardiac failure.

It would seem therefore that the interest of these symptoms lies not so much in the persisting disability they cause, nor in the problems of management they pose in the acute stage after injury, but more in the fact that they reflect the frequency with which some damage is sustained by the hypothalamus in severe closed head injury. Of particular interest is the common association in the present study of hyperphagia in the early stages of recovery from injury and the release of irritability, often amounting to the 'sham rage' of experimentally decorticated animals, which persists as a permanent personality change. It seems reasonable to propose that lesions situated in similar areas and interrupting cortical and hypothalamic connections which release the physiological concomitants of rage in the experimental animal might be the same as those responsible for the persisting irritability so common after severe closed head injury.

9 Systemic Complications and Peripheral Nerve, Bone and Joint Injury

This chapter deals both with those disabilities persisting in the long-term which have arisen as a result of injury to structures apart from the brain and cranial nerves, and also with those systemic disorders other than the metabolic ones already considered. There is no detailed review of the extent to which these complications contributed to the problems of rehabilitation in the survivors who were re-examined, although this was often substantial, since the principal aim of this investigation was the assessment of long-term outcome after severe trauma to the central nervous system. Attempts to assess the time sequence of recovery of the central neural lesions were complicated by the presence of long bone fractures, despite the fact that they played a small part in eventual disability.

Rather than exclude every patient with femoral and tibial shaft fractures from the sequential assessment of central neural grades of disability, it seemed justifiable to examine each case in detail, and by making comparisons with other patients whose neural lesions were similar, but who had not sustained leg fractures, to attempt an estimate of neural disability assuming the injury had not been complicated by the immobilisation necessitated by these fractures. In most cases it was possible to assign a disability grade at certain selected intervals after injury on the basis of the neural lesions described in the case notes, which allowed an assumption that the patient would have been walking by then were it not for his leg injuries. This was a simple matter when the head injury resulted either in relatively trivial or in very severe neural lesions. When difficulties in making the assessment arose, none was attempted, and the patient was excluded from the computer-assisted analysis of the rate of recovery as a predictor of final outcome (described in chapter 13).

Hypoxia, Hypotension, Gut, Renal and Chest Complications

The effects of systemic hypoxia or hypotension and secondary cerebral perfusion failure were not examined specifically but, as discussed in an earlier chapter, these undoubtedly contributed to the deterioration in the neurological state of many patients after admission to hospital. The effect this had on the final outcome has already been described. Even amongst the survivors a variety of other forms of systemic complication were observed, including a number of cases of intestinal haemorrhage, gastric atony and paralytic ileus, a few in which temporary renal failure, and many in which renal infection gave rise to problems of management in the acute stage after injury. There were many more in which chest infection complicated the first few post-traumatic days or weeks. The only patient with a gastrointestinal complication which continued to give trouble years later was a woman with achalasia of the oesophagus which had declared itself in a minor form before the injury. Long-term renal problems were seen in only three patients. The first was a boy whose injuries included rupture of the urethra with subsequent stenosis. This caused hydronephrosis requiring repeated surgical procedures over many years. The second was a young man whose prolonged decubitus, resulting from the head injury, caused stag-horn renal calculi and subsequent hypertension. One patient developed acute glomerulonephritis shortly after injury, which was proven by biopsy 2 years later and left some permanent impairment of renal function. There were two adolescents whose convalescence after prolonged coma was protracted by the development of pulmonary tuberculosis, and another who required a segmental lobectomy for bronchiectasis 18 months after her injury. In none of these cases was the head injury certainly responsible for the pulmonary complications, although it may have been contributory in all.

It was clear from the death certificates and hospital records examined that systemic complications, particularly chest and renal infection, and also venous thrombosis and decubitus ulcers, were wholly or partially responsible for the deaths of the 103 patients who failed to recover from their head injuries sufficiently to be discharged from hospital. It is probable, as discussed in chapter 12 on life expectancy, that chest infection contributed to the premature deaths of a number of demented patients confined to psychiatric institutions or geriatric homes. There was no evidence of continuing disability due to these various complications of the head injury in the remaining survivors examined.

Meningitis

As a complication of the acute stage this had excluded a number of patients from the study. Amongst the survivors in both series of patients examined, there was only one case in which meningitis developed for the first time in convalescence after discharge. This was a boy of five whose streptococcal meningitis occurred 5 weeks after his accident whilst in the hospital to which he had been returned. It was attributed to an infected burr hole. A girl of fifteen at the time her head injury had caused a comminuted parietal fracture extending into the petrous and bleeding from an ear, developed her first attack of pneumococcal meningitis 3 years later, and her second 5 years later, having otherwise made an excellent recovery from her head injury. Repair of the dural tear in the middle fossa after her second attack prevented any recurrence in the succeeding 11 years. Reference will be made in chapter 12 to the three patients who died 1, 2 and 4 years after injury from pneumococcal meningitis acquired via middle and anterior cranial fossa fractures.

Peripheral Nerve Injury

There were a small number of radial and ulnar nerve palsies recorded in the case notes, and a rather larger number of common peroneal palsies, the latter apparently due either to decubitus or to local injury often associated with fractures in the lower leg. There was no patient with persisting disability due to a peripheral nerve lesion in the arm, even in the case of one who had developed myositis ossificans in an arm partially paralysed by a radial palsy. In only one ambulant patient was there persisting evidence of a common peroneal palsy. He had sustained multiple injuries including compound fractures of the tibia and fibula and traumatic section of a number of ankle tendons. The generally benign outlook for these closed peripheral nerve lesions associated with head injuries in civilian life is in keeping with the observations of Seddon (1972) and Sunderland (1972). In striking contrast are the persisting disabilities resulting from closed avulsion injuries of the brachial plexus. In this study, again because it is principally concerned with brain injury, all patients recorded as having brachial plexus lesions on the punchcards were excluded. However, one patient was written to by mistake and asked to attend for examination. In a motor-cycle accident 13 years previously he had sustained a complete brachial plexus avulsion, in addition to the head injury which had been severe enough to cause coma lasting for a month. He has been excluded from the study but it seems worth commenting on the fact that his mild brainstem cerebellar syndrome, defective memory and slight frontal personality change seemed trivial disabilities by comparison with the persistently painful phantom arm resulting from his peripheral injuries.

Skeletal Injuries

All patients recorded as having spinal cord damage had been excluded from the follow-up study. Two re-examined patients who had not had radiological evidence of injury to the vertebral column and who, at the time, were not considered to have sustained spinal cord damage, were found to have severe spastic parapareses in incomplete extension. In each case there were also profound personality changes suggesting considerable frontal lobe injury on both sides, but there was not the severe pseudobulbar pattern of lesions more usually seen with these degrees of paraplegia. This raised the possibility of spinal cord contusion, but in neither case could this be certainly confirmed. A small number of other patients without any sign of spinal cord injury had radiological evidence of fractures of vertebral spines or transverse processes. These did not have any notable long-term effects, any more than the fractured ribs, scapulae or clavicles which complicated many head injuries.

There were 31 patients (11 per cent) in the consecutive series, and 11 (17 per cent) in the selected series, whose injuries included fractures of femoral or tibial shafts. The ages at the time of injury and the bones involved are

recorded in table 9.1. It was most striking that despite head injury severe
enough to cause post-traumatic amnesia exceeding a week in every case,
fractures of the femur were more frequently the principal cause of prolonged
convalescence and delay in return to work than the sequelae of the head

Table 9.1   Fractures of femur and/or tibia, and fractures of tibia without femoral
fracture

	Ages		
	5–25 years	26–45 years	46 years+
Consecutive series			
Uncomplicated			
Total patients	214		
Number with fractured femoral shaft(s)	13	8	5
Percentage	6%		(2 femoral necks)
Number with fractured tibial shaft(s)	10	6	2	2
Percentage	5%		
Complicated			
Total patients	77		
Number with fractured femoral shaft(s)	0	0	0	0
Percentage	0%		
Number with fractured tibial shaft(s)	8	3	4	1
Percentage	11%		
Selected series			
Total patients	64		
Number with fractured femoral shaft(s)	5	5	0	0
Percentage	8%		
Number with fractured tibial shaft(s)	6	5	1	0
Percentage	9%		

injury. Indeed, many patients with fractures of the femur or tibia, when asked
to recall the disabilities resulting from their head injuries, were able only to
describe the long period of plaster immobilisation and their defective balance.
Only in patients whose brain injury resulted in severe persisting central neural
disability did it appear that fractures of the femur were of less importance in
physical rehabilitation in the short-term than the effects of head injury. It was
equally clear that, in the long-term, personality change and memory impairment, even in the absence of more than marginal evidence of central neural
lesions, were more serious persisting sequelae of the accident than a limp due
to slight shortening of a leg.

There were 49 patients from the consecutive series, and 17 from the selected, that is 17 per cent and 27 per cent respectively, whose head injuries had been complicated by fractures of the long bones of one or both arms, or fractures of the clavicle. This had resulted in a proportion of patients with some long-term disability due to an incomplete range of movement at one or more joints, but this was rarely the subject of complaint and in not one case did this constitute the main, or indeed any significant, disability.

Neurogenic Para-articular Ossification

Myositis ossificans was noted and abstracted from the case notes of six patients amongst the re-examined survivors. In each case coma had lasted for a month or more. In one there was no clinical evidence of any reduction in the range of movement at the joints involved. In another, examined 8 years after injury, who had made a good recovery from his central neural lesions, convalescence had been complicated by severe myositis ossificans of both hips and knees, and finally bony ankylosis of the hips. This had persisted and was his main disability apart from that due to a moderate frontal personality change and defective day-to-day memory. There was also some slight restriction of the range of movement of both his knees. The four other cases were all still severely disabled by spastic paresis of the legs, and in all of these movements at the hips and knees and in one an arm as well remained greatly restricted, presumably by bony ankylosis. Radiological evidence to confirm this was not available at the time of the follow-up study.

Cerebral Fat Emboli

This diagnosis was made on the basis of the appearance of petechial haemorrhages of the skin or retina in four patients from the consecutive series whose injuries had been complicated by femoral or tibial fractures. In two of these it seemed possible, in view of the almost total absence of neurophysical disability in the presence of extensor plantar responses in the one and the absence of abnormal neural signs in the other, that this systemic complication of the head injury, rather than the cerebral effects of trauma or cerebral perfusion failure, had been the cause of the deterioration in their neurological states in the acute stage after injury.

Discussion

It is self-evident that the secondary systemic complications of hypoxia, hypotension and fat embolism due to multiple injuries often contribute to the brain damage which occurs in head injury. The extent to which they do so has not been examined in any detail in this study. It is certain that cerebral infarction can, and often does, cause more extensive and more disabling permanent sequelae than those due to acceleration shear strains, but it is by no means clear in which cases this is so. Moreover, systemic hypoxia and hypotension associated with chest injury and airways obstruction, or due to fractures of major long bones, are potentially reversible given appropriate treatment, whereas nothing will alter damage done to the brain by mechanical forces acting at the moment of impact. Yet even the treatment of skeletal injuries may provide a final disastrous insult to the already damaged brain. The effects of general anaesthesia in raising intracranial pressure and reducing cerebral perfusion have been examined by McDowall, Barker and Jennett (1966), and this potential hazard of general anaesthesia in head injury has been discussed by Jennett (1970). In this study it has only been possible to refer in passing to these complex contributory factors to long-term disability after severe head injury. It has been simple, by contrast, to assess the contribution to long-term disability made by certain skeletal injuries and myositis ossificans, by the acute pulmonary, renal and gastrointestinal complications and by associated peripheral nerve injury and late meningeal infection.

Meningitis as a late sequel to skull fracture was, with a single exception, confined to fractures involving the floor of the middle cranial fossa in the five cases found in the consecutive series. This seems likely to reflect the active attitude to surgical treatment of fractures of the anterior fossa and paranasal sinuses taken by Lewin (1966) in his management of these patients. These figures cannot, unfortunately, be taken as a fully reliable estimate of meningitis complicating head injury after an interval of time since, if this interval were short, meningitis would have been entered on the punchcard and the patient excluded from the follow-up study. The observation does, however, provide further support for the views of, amongst others, Jefferson and Reilly (1972), on the importance of surgical treatment for fractures extending into the floor of the anterior fossa, and raises again the question of the need for prophylactic antibiotics in cases where it appears that there may be fractures extending into the petrous, even when this has not been certainly confirmed.

The management of long bone fractures of the legs in these patients has been described by Gibson (1960). Definitive treatment was often delayed in cases where the severity of the head injury appeared to justify it. The early results have been mentioned briefly by Lewin (1966). Despite the problems posed by delirium, hypertonus and decerebration, internal fixation as advocated by Glenn, Miner and Peltier (1973) was not used. Its obvious advantages were considered insufficient to counterbalance both the dangers of further operative procedures in the severely head-injured, and the risks of wound infection in incontinent and restless patients. Amongst the survivors the end results were the same whether definitive treatment took place within a few hours or was delayed for several days. The long-term results observed in the present study were excellent in that disability due to minor shortening and deformity appeared to be minimal although, admittedly, this could not be judged accurately in those severely disabled by their neural lesions. By contrast, the problems posed in the short-term rehabilitation of patients with severe joint and long bone injury were often considerable, and when combined with severe neural disabilities they stretched the resources of rehabilitation centres over a period of many months and in some cases of years. This subject has been well reviewed by Vigouroux and his colleagues in their publication already referred to (Vigouroux *et al.*, 1972), and is not dealt with further here.

There seems to have been no previous examination of the long-term outlook for the phenomenon of neurogenic para-articular ossification amongst survivors of severe head injury. It is not clear from the account given by Vigouroux and his colleagues what proportion of the 10 per cent of their patients who suffered coma lasting longer than 3 weeks and who developed this complication were still disabled by the effects of heterotopic calcification many years later. It seems that, as with the para-articular ossifications associated with the spinal cord injuries reviewed by Guttmann (1976), where there is recovery of the voluntary control of the limbs, there is normally rapid resorption of the abnormal bone. The fact that this is not always the case is demonstrated by the one patient examined for this study 8 years after his injury, whose neural disabilities were mild but whose hips remained permanently ankylosed despite all efforts. Whether early treatment with disodium etidronate, had it been available, since shown to be helpful in myositis ossificans progressiva by Russell, Smith, Bishop, Price and Squire (1972), might have affected the long-term outcome in this uncommon type of case, remains to be seen.

There is no information available (of which the author is aware) describing the long-term effects of cerebral fat embolisation complicating long bone fractures. Sevitt (1960) has underlined the fact that even massive pulmonary fat embolisation is a relatively benign phenomenon, this also being so in the short-term even when there has been systemic and cerebral embolism. In two of the four cases with clinical evidence of fat emboli whose neurological state deteriorated substantially after admission to hospital, there was no disability attributable to neural lesions in the long-term despite the presence of extensor plantar responses in one patient. It is possible that it is not the petechial haemorrhages – on the evidence presented by Hoare (1971) the result of intimal damage by irritant fatty acids released from fat globules – and thrombocytopenia, which are responsible for permanent neural disability in the survivors of fat embolism. Rather it could be due to cerebral perfusion failure secondary to hypoxia and the systemic hypotensive effects of the multiple injuries.

10 Prevalence and Natural History of Post-traumatic Epilepsy

In all there were 75 patients amongst the 291 comprising the consecutive series, examined between 10 and 24 years after their injuries, who were found to have had one or more post-traumatic epileptic attacks, and who had not previously been subject to epilepsy. In addition there were four amongst the 178 dead from this series who had died as a result of their traumatic epilepsy. Except in so far as epilepsy had been a cause of death, information was incomplete about the incidence of epilepsy amongst the dead. Therefore no attempt will be made to assess the overall incidence and prevalence amongst the entire 469, that is living and dead, traced in the consecutive series. Apart from its effect on life expectancy, this study of the prevalence and natural history of post-traumatic epilepsy is confined to the survivors who were re-examined.

The post-traumatic epileptic attack or attacks were confined to the first week after injury in 22 of these 75 patients. In 17 the injury was uncomplicated and in the remaining five complicated by surface brain compression with or without traumatic or surgical brain penetration. In 15 patients the attacks were limited to one or more, and seldom more than half a dozen focal motor seizures, a few progressing to generalised convulsions. In the remainder there was usually a single, or again, less than half a dozen generalised convulsions without focal onset. These patients, whose epileptic attacks ceased after the first week will not be considered further, except briefly when the question of 'early' epilepsy occurring in the first week after injury is examined as a factor predicting the likelihood of 'late' post-traumatic epilepsy developing thereafter.

In the remaining 53 patients who did have further attacks after the first week the relationship between their epilepsy and type of head injury, incidence of skull fracture, and severity of the injury, as judged by the length of post-traumatic amnesia and duration of coma, is examined in tables 10.1, 10.2 and 10.3. It can be seen that cerebral compression due to subdural or extradural bleeding or hygroma, which is associated with polar contusion, laceration or swelling requiring surgical internal decompression, carries the risk of post-traumatic epilepsy developing in 61 per cent of cases. Traumatic brain penetration without brain compression carries a very similar risk, although surgical brain penetration for the removal of necrotic temporal or frontal poles, at 43 per cent, has a somewhat lower risk.

It is also apparent that with increasing severity of the injury, judged by these two indirect measures of 'diffuse brain concussion', duration of post-traumatic amnesia and coma, there is a trend towards increasing prevalence of post-traumatic epilepsy, but this is minimal compared with the effects of brain penetration.

Table 10.1 Prevalence of late and early epilepsy related to type of complication of the injury

	Uncomplicated	Complicated†	Complicated			
			Surface brain compression alone	Compression with brain penetration surgical or traumatic (only one traumatic)	Traumatic brain penetration without compression	Surgical brain penetration for debridement and internal compression
Patient totals	214	77	39	13	14	7
Late epilepsy						
Number	24	29	10	8	8	3
Percentage	10%	38%	26%	61%	57%	43%
Early epilepsy						
Number	5	5	2	3	0	0
Fractured skull						
Number	17	27	9	8	8	3
Percentage	85%	93%	90%	100%	100%	100%

Consecutive series, total 291 patients.   † Includes 4 additional cases in which complication was vascular: arterial or sinus thrombosis

Table 10.2 Late traumatic epilepsy, duration of PTA and incidence of skull fracture in uncomplicated injury

| | | Weeks PTA | |
	1 week	1–3 weeks	4 weeks +
Patient totals	61	82	51
Number with epilepsy	5	11	8
Percentage with epilepsy	7%	14%	16%
Number with skull fracture	5	6	6

Consecutive series, total 291 patients.

Table 10.3 Late traumatic epilepsy, duration of coma, and complication of injury

	Duration of coma			
	1 month or longer		Less than 1 month	
	Total number of patients			
	64		267	
	Complicated	Uncomplicated	Complicated	Uncomplicated
Totals	23	41	67	200
Number with epilepsy	10	7	25	22
Percentage with epilepsy	43%	17%	37%	11%

Selected and consecutive series, total 331 patients.

The severity of the post-traumatic epilepsy, the type of clinical attack and the association with the type of head injury are noted in table 10.4. Injuries complicated by brain penetration, surface compression, or both are more likely to give rise to focal motor attacks, with or without progression to major convulsions, than are uncomplicated injuries. These, conversely, give rise to a higher proportion of generalised convulsions without focal onset. Statistically the attacks are no more severe or disabling whether they succeed a complicated or uncomplicated injury, but numbers are small and there is a trend towards more frequent attacks after complicated injuries. The tabulation also obscures the fact that more patients with uncomplicated injuries who had fewer than half a dozen attacks a year, had in fact only experienced one or two isolated attacks, usually during the first year after injury; those with complicated injuries, on the other hand, tended to have rather more attacks, although still less than six a year. In addition this analysis also fails to record the potentially serious single episode of epileptic status or serial convulsions, and the fact that two patients with infrequent fits sustained a second severe head injury in isolated attacks. There were three patients whose minor temporal lobe attacks caused no inconvenience. They had remained undiagnosed and untreated since the injury. One of them also had a homonymous hemianopia. Neither of his disabilities had prevented him from driving ammunition lorries for many years after his injury.

Table 10.4   Severity of 'late' post-traumatic epilepsy related to complication and type of clinical attack

	Uncomplicated		Complicated	
	Few attacks	6 or more a year	Few attacks	6 or more a year
Totals				
Consecutive	17	7	18	11
Selected	(5)*		(6)*	
Focal motor† (⅓ Jacksonian in both complicated and un-complicated injuries)	4 (1)*	1	10 (4)*	4 (1 intractable)
Temporal lobe epilepsy (½ minor aura, ¼ automatisms or convulsions; in both complicated and uncomplicated in-juries)	3 (1)*	3	3	4
Generalised convulsions without focal onset (some noc-turnal)	10 (3)*	3 (1 intractable) (1 solely nocturnal)	5 (2)*	3 (1 intractable)

Consecutive and selected series, total 331 patients.

* Patients from selected series.

† Patients have been included here when any of the attacks were focal in onset, although the majority may have been major convulsions without focal onset.

In injuries complicated by surface compression, but without brain penetration – either traumatic, or surgical for the removal of lacerated and swollen brain tissue – the incidence of post-traumatic epilepsy declines to something less than 30 per cent. In injuries which have not been complicated a slight increase in prevalence is seen with increasing duration of post-traumatic amnesia, despite a decreasing incidence of skull fracture.

The *natural history* of the late post-traumatic epilepsy in these 53 patients is shown graphically in figure 10.1 against a semilogarithmic time-scale. Each

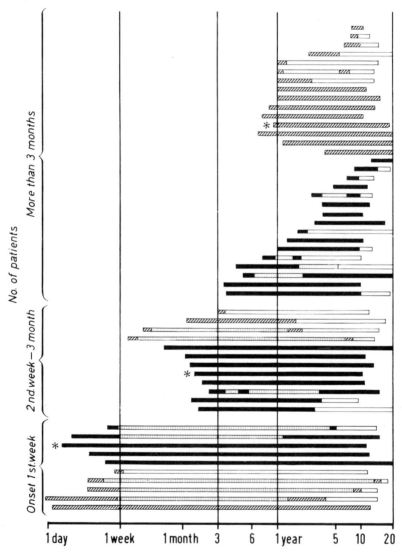

Figure 10.1   Post-traumatic epilepsy. The three cases in which the patients were severely disabled by frequent major fits are indicated by asterisks. ■ Complicated 29 (38 per cent); ▥ uncomplicated 24 (9 per cent); □ remission; ▨ incomplete remission.

patient is represented by a single line, and these are grouped to highlight the relationships between times of onset, separately, for the complicated and uncomplicated injuries and also the type and duration of remission. Only in the three cases starred could the epilepsy be considered seriously disabling in that frequent major attacks continued despite all attempts at treatment short of surgery. In table 10.5 the number of patients whose epilepsy remitted

Table 10.5   Late traumatic epilepsy in relation to age at injury and 'complete' remission

	Age at injury		
	5–15 years	16–35 years	36 years +
Total number of patients	48	153	90
Number with epilepsy	10	28	15
Percentage with epilepsy	21%	19%	16%
'Complete' remission from 3–17 years	6	14	5
Percentage having 'complete' remission	60%	50%	33%

Consecutive complicated and uncomplicated series, total 291 patients.

'completely' is examined in relation to age at time of injury. Remission was reckoned to be 'complete' if there had been no attacks of any kind for over 3 years. In fact, of these 25 patients whose fits had ceased, 17 had not had an attack for over 5 years by the time of follow-up and the remaining eight had been free of fits for over 3 years. There had been a long delay before this more permanent remission set in. In the case of 14 patients it was 5 years after the injury before they finally achieved remission, for another seven patients 10 years and in the case of one further patient, 15 years. The fact that this last patient had been free of fits for the 15 years before his last single attack draws attention to the uncertainties involved in assuming permanent remission where the period of follow-up has been shorter than is the case here. In the majority of patients, both those who finally achieved remission and those who did not, the frequency of focal and non-focal convulsions declined to negligible numbers over the years. In the fifth of the patients who finally remitted there were long periods of 'temporary' remission extending over many years, which were then followed by an isolated attack, or, in some cases, two or three attacks, before the 'final' remission.

In the consecutive series of patients there had been 31 who had experienced one or more epileptic attacks in the first week after injury. In the case of 10 of these the epilepsy had subsequently recurred. In five this took a remarkably benign form, with one further fit and thereafter complete remission for 16 years in the case of one patient, whilst in the remaining five there were many years of freedom from attacks followed by one or two fits and then remission again. The risk of post-traumatic epilepsy recurring following attacks in the first week after injury was about one in three compared with one in six for the rest of the consecutive series who had not had fits in the first week.

The Electroencephalogram

Electroencephalograms had not been recorded routinely for every patient included in this study. Indeed, even in the case of patients who developed post-traumatic epilepsy following their discharge from hospital, this was often after a substantial interval, and where a diagnosis was made, investigations were in many cases carried out elsewhere so that records were not available at the Radcliffe Infirmary. There were no facilities for repeating the records when the patients were re-examined for the study. Electroencephalograms were not recorded for eight patients with epilepsy of the 29 in the consecutive series whose injuries had been complicated, nor for eight of the 24 whose injuries were uncomplicated. Moreover, recordings were not made at any set interval after head injury, but rather when clinical management or the special interests of the surgeon suggested the need. All the records were made post-operatively in patients who developed epilepsy in association with complicated injuries. Many more recordings were made of patients whose traumatic epilepsy continued to present a problem in management than in cases where it did not.

It was therefore not possible to examine the predictive value of the electroencephalogram for the development of post-traumatic epilepsy in this series of patients, nor the value which it might or might not have had in indicating which patients who developed epilepsy were likely to be disabled by it or in which cases remission was likely to occur.

In table 10.6 a comparison is drawn between the clinical and electroencephalographic type of epilepsy in both complicated and uncomplicated

Table 10.6   Clinical and electroencephalographic type of epilepsy

	Clinical attacks		EEG abnormality	
Total number of patients	53	Number with EEG records*	37	(21 complicated, 4 uncomplicated injuries)
Focal sensorimotor	19	Total focal	27	(2 more than one focus)
Percentage	36%		76%	
Temporal lobe epilepsy	13	TL focus	8	(6 complicated, 2 uncomplicated injuries)
Percentage	24%		23%	
Generalised convulsions without focal onset	21	Non-focal or indifinite foci	10	
Percentage	40%		27%	

Consecutive series, total 291 patients.
* The relatively small number here reflects the fact that many developed their epilepsy some time after discharge from hospital, and were seen elsewhere for the epilepsy and its investigation. Three cases remained undiagnosed until seen for this study.

injuries. The substantially higher prevalence of focal epilepsy with electro-physiological evidence after complicated injury is apparent, as is also the greater frequency of its temporal lobe variant. This is despite the suggestion, from the clinical evidence alone, that post-traumatic temporal lobe epilepsy is equally prevalent after uncomplicated and complicated injury. The higher proportion of focal epilepsies after complicated injuries, together with low incidence after uncomplicated injuries, and also the fact that many more patients have early epilepsy which does not recur after uncomplicated injury, suggests differing aetiologies. This seems to be at least partially true and provides some evidence for constitutional predisposition causing temporary failure of inhibitory mechanisms, rather than that all post-traumatic epilepsy originates in focal brain damage.

The relationship between side of head impact and the focal EEG abnormality noted in the earliest recording made is examined in table 10.7. In this

Table 10.7   Side of head impact and side of earliest EEG voltage attenuation and/or focal slow wave abnormality

| | Focal EEG abnormality | |
	ipsilateral	contralateral
Uncomplicated injury		
Total number of patients 39*		
Number with lateralised EEG abnormality	14	25
Percentage	36%	64%
Complicated injury		
Total number of patients 32*		
Number with lateralised EEG abnormality	21	11
Percentage	66%	34%

Consecutive series, total 291 patients.
*Number of patients among those with EEG records which showed a focal abnormality and in whom it was possible to identify the side of head impact.

focal or lateralised suppression of electrical activity, or attenuation of voltage, was considered the side of major brain injury. Where there was no voltage suppression a slow wave focus was recorded as the site of damage. Generalised abnormalities, even when asymmetrical, were not included in this analysis. It may be seen that, as in the clinical assessment, there is evidence of contre-coup brain damage in uncomplicated head injuries.

Discussion

The findings in this study accord well with those of Jennett and Lewin (1960) and with Jennett (1962, 1969, 1975), as well they might since the earliest of the above papers was based on data derived from a study of the first 1000 consecutive cases of the 7000 from which the present series of patients has more recently been taken. In patients who had an epileptic attack in the first week after their injuries these authors found that rather less than one in three developed 'late' epilepsy, having further fits after the first week. In the present study a similar proportion, 10 of the 31 who had early epilepsy, had later epileptic attacks. By contrast, in the present study there is an overall prevalence of late epilepsy amongst those who did not have an early fit of one in six, that is 44 out of 260 patients. This is substantially higher than the one in ten found by Jennett and Lewin who followed their patients for 4 years. The present study included a larger proportion of severe injuries, and also of patients requiring internal decompression for cerebral lacerations. There were also differences in the classification of complications used in the two studies. The principal concern here has been the assessment of long-term neurological disability in relation to measures of severity of injury. In attempting to establish those characteristics of the injury which were more likely than others to be associated with disability, it was felt that a distinction should be made between penetration of brain substance and simple dural penetration. In most cases surgery for the removal of necrotic brain, with or without associated intracerebral haematomata, was the form taken by brain penetration. Patients whose injuries were not complicated by surgical or traumatic brain penetration, even if found at operation to require dural repair, were classified as having uncomplicated injuries. This applied also, for similar reasons, in the case of patients who were submitted to exploratory burr holes which failed to reveal subdural bleeding sufficient to cause brain compression. In fact, seven of the latter patients developed late epilepsy, as did one six-year-old boy who required elevation of a depressed fracture over the frontal cortex which, like the dura, remained intact. If the figures for the prevalence of late epilepsy are adjusted to include this boy and three other patients with traumatic dural – but not brain – penetration, who did not develop epilepsy, there is no material change in the prevalence figures. At 61 per cent the figure for brain penetration and surface compression in combination is higher than that for acute subdural haematoma reported by Jennett, and approximates to that for the combination of dural penetration, early epilepsy and post-traumatic amnesia lasting longer than 24 hours found in a large series of patients with depressed skull fractures by Jennett, Miller and Braakman (1974), and by Grob and Ketz (1974). The latter authors draw attention to the fact that actual 'leakage of brain substance' increases the risk of epilepsy developing from 33 per cent with dural penetration only, to 45 per cent. The figure of 61 per cent is also higher than the 48 per cent noted for intracerebral haematomas by Jennett (1975), and the overall prevalence after brain-penetrating missile wounds of all grades of severity in three wars which, in each, was in the region of 40 per cent, according to Caviness (1969), Russell and Whitty (1952) and Walker and Jablon (1961).

In the present study severity of the 'diffuse' brain concussion, measured indirectly by duration of post-traumatic amnesia and coma, was found to increase the prevalence of late epilepsy in both complicated and uncomplicated injuries, but this was relatively slight where the risks were already high.

It was Jennett's conclusion, stated in his monograph (Jennett, 1962), that since there were so many severely affected, and for many years, it was unwise to assume that the complication of post-traumatic epilepsy once it appeared, would be either mild or temporary. He pointed out, however, that his study had been biased towards the more severely disabling forms of traumatic epilepsy. This was so because his patients tended to be gathered from colleagues seeking advice in cases which posed problems in management. He made no claim, therefore, that his data could be used to indicate what proportion of all cases of traumatic epilepsy were likely to be severely disabling in the long-term. Only 79 of his 198 patients were followed for longer than 10 years, and this, although a larger overall number than in the present study, is a smaller proportion of his total series in which the long-term natural history has been studied. All the patients in the consecutive series in the present investigation were followed for longer than 10 years, and since only 10 patients from the entire consecutive series remained untraced, it may reasonably be assumed that the evidence for the generally benign long-term character of post-traumatic epilepsy after closed head injuries is established. This becomes increasingly apparent only over the course of many years: epileptic attacks not only became progressively less frequent in the case of all but three patients in the consecutive series who were re-examined, but in the majority of cases the attacks also became abortive or minor variants of the earlier ones. In 15 patients it would not have been possible, earlier than 10 years after injury, to assume that a remission lasting longer than 3 years was going to take place. These observations are in keeping with the long-term prospects for epilepsy after brain-penetrating missile wounds reported by both Walker and Erculei (1970) and by Russell and Davies-Jones (1969). It must, however, be conceded that in the case of four patients premature deaths were directly related to traumatic epilepsy in the consecutive series, and there were two patients among the survivors, both with infrequent fits, who suffered second severe head injuries as a result of isolated attacks.

Whether late epilepsy would become disabling or persist only in a benign form was, as Caveness (1963) has shown for missile wounds, very closely related to the frequency and character of the attacks in the individual case. Although it was not possible to identify at an early stage patients whose epilepsy, when it developed, was going to be intractable or disabling, those who had once developed late fits which recurred with any frequency continued to present with management problems, whereas infrequent attacks, on the other hand, became less frequent. In other words, as in the case of disseminated sclerosis, prediction became possible and then accurate only after late epilepsy had been observable over a period of time. The three intractable cases all started within a year of injury, but they otherwise had exhibited no distinguishing features which would have suggested that these particular patients were going to be the ones severely disabled.

This study contributes little to any further understanding of the mechanisms which provoke epilepsy after head injury or of how these affect the long-term prognosis. It has confirmed the well-recognised fact that brain penetration is the most important factor, and adds support to the suggestion that increasingly severe diffuse 'concussive' injury superimposed upon this, will further increase the risks to some variable extent. It is not clear from Jennett and his colleagues' observations on epilepsy after non-missile head injury with depressed skull fracture how far brain penetration, rather than contusion through intact or merely torn dura, increases the prevalence. The suggestion first made by Russell and Whitty (1952) that it is a combination of damage to cortex and deep subcortical pathways concerned in the physiological inhibition of widespread neuronal discharges is certainly supported by the highest incidence amongst patients with burst temporal lobes and surface compression. A necrotic temporal pole, lacerated, haemorrhagic, and requiring internal decompression, while in itself highly likely to give rise to late epilepsy, becomes even more liable to do so when associated surface brain compression has caused secondary infarction at other sites. These, characteristically, are the highly epileptogenic mesial temporal areas. When the focal injury has been relatively less severe, without brain penetration or compression, and even when diffuse injury has been substantial, measured by long post-traumatic amnesia, there is a higher incidence of early epilepsy amongst patients with uncomplicated injuries who do not develop 'late' epilepsy. This suggests constitutional predisposition. The head injury in these cases merely seems to have provided the adequate provocation in those predisposed to have fits by a relatively lower threshold.

In none of his more recent papers has Jennett confirmed the remarkably high prevalence of post-traumatic epilepsy of 80 per cent reported in his monograph for patients with depressed fractures, dural penetration and post-traumatic amnesia lasting longer than 24 hours. It is probable that these unusual risks reflected his small number of patients with this combination of features. Only with brain penetration and infection does the prevalence normally rise to these levels, which are characteristic of the rates after intracranial abscesses, at 70 per cent, reported by Legg, Gupta and Scott (1973). The inconstant relationship between the prevalence of post-traumatic epilepsy and the well-recognised histological sequelae of trauma have been the subject of review repeatedly over the past 50 years, amongst others, by Penfield (1927), Courville (1958), Rasmussen (1969) and Payan, Toga and Bérard-Badier (1970). No generally satisfying explanation has been put forward for the way in which these permanent histological changes result, in the majority of cases, in a gradual decrease with time in the severity and frequency of the various forms of post-traumatic epileptic attacks for which they are held responsible. Apart from reiterating this remarkable fact, and confirming that the long-term natural history of epilepsy following either severe blunt accidental or missile-penetrating brain injury is identical, the evidence collected in this study does no more than underline the present state of ignorance of the neurophysiology of traumatic epilepsy.

11 Progressive Post-traumatic Encephalopathy and Premature Ageing

It was a particular purpose of this study to attempt to establish whether or not there was a condition which might properly be described as progressive post-traumatic encephalopathy. The earlier study by the author of the late effects of repeated minor head injuries in a random sample of ex-professional boxers had confirmed that this did occur in a small proportion of cases, but the very slowly progressing impairment of intellectual functions and personality exhibited by the majority of the boxers who had deteriorated later in life seemed most likely to be attributable to the effects of normal ageing superimposed upon an already damaged brain. With this evidence that repeated minor injury to the brain did seem, rarely, to be capable of producing a condition that would cause progressive damage long after the trauma had ceased, but that in most cases late deterioration was almost certainly due to the exaggerated effects of ageing, a detailed examination of these two possible explanations of progressive and late deterioration after a single injury seemed worthwhile. Every patient was questioned at length to elicit his own observations about increasing difficulties with memory, learning, expressing himself and job performance. In each case the relative was similarly asked for her observations of the spouse's intellectual function over the years since the injury, and of any late changes in personality or behaviour.

Among the survivors re-examined, those patients for whom there was some evidence, however slight, of either progressive deterioration in intellectual functions, personality and behaviour or of neural disabilities are described briefly in table 11.1. It may be seen that in cases 1–10 the question of a progressive dementing process arises. In two cases this had developed in the senium, and in the remaining eight in the presenium as this is conventionally accepted. Case 1 presented with an acute paranoid delusional psychosis some months after his discharge from hospital. A poor response to treatment and the continuing threats he made to kill his wife led to his permanent commitment to a psychiatric hospital 3 years after his injury. He had had frequent generalised convulsions since late adolescence and the head injury was a sequel to one of these. The attacks remained poorly controlled and continued at the rate of more than a dozen a year. The electroencephalogram showed a temporal lobe focus and his progressive dementia and schizophrenia-like psychosis seem likely to have been due to repeated anoxic damage caused by his epilepsy, superimposed upon relatively minor brain injury, rather than to the injury itself. In case 2 the injury, judged by the permanent dementia it caused, was of considerably greater severity. The patient was a heavy drinking

Table 11.1 Patients with progressing dementia and/or neural disabilities since the head injury

Sex and series number	Age at injury	Age examined	Duration PTA and complication	Nature of progressive deterioration and pattern of neural lesions
Case 1, male C82, consecutive	35	49	2 weeks; extradural clot	Paranoid delusional psychosis 3 months after with increasing frequency pre-traumatic major fits. Progressive dementia thereafter. Permanent in-patient mental hospital 8 years. Brainstem cerebellar syndrome.
Case 2, male S18, consecutive	46	65	Permanent; uncomplicated	Post-traumatic Korzakow state, then chronic paranoid delusional symptomatology in setting of progressive dementia and alcoholism complicated by adequately controlled post-traumatic epilepsy. Permanent in-patient mental hospital 17 years. Brainstem cerebellar syndrome.
Case 3, male S94, consecutive	32	47	4 weeks; uncomplicated	Slowly progressive paranoid dementia 8 years. Pre-traumatic temporal lobe epilepsy adequately controlled. Cared for by brother. Unclassifiable pattern of neural lesions.
Case 4, female S222, consecutive	62	76	Permanent; uncomplicated	Post-traumatic dementia static 7 years progressing rapidly 3 years. Cared for by sister. Neural lesions unclassifiable.
Case 5, male S36, consecutive	44	65	5 weeks; uncomplicated	Slowly progressive paranoid dementia in last 6 years. Recurrent endogenous depressions before and since. Cared for by wife. Mild brainstem cerebellar pattern.
Case 6, male C48, consecutive	43	59	3 months; acute subdural clot then hygroma	Improvement first 8 years then slowly progressive dementia. Cared for by wife. Mild hemiparetic pattern.
Case 7, male C115, consecutive	63	75	7 weeks; acute subdural clot and hygroma	Slowly progressive dementia since. Cared for by wife. Minimal hemiparetic pattern.

Case				
Case 8, male C120, consecutive	45	66	6 weeks; traumatic dural brain penetration	Progressive dementia since 2 years after injury. Cared for by wife. Mild hemiparetic pattern.
Case 9, male S258, consecutive	71	86	Permanent; uncomplicated	Progressively dementing since. Cared for by grand-daughter. Unclassifiable pattern neural lesions.
Case 10, male S71, consecutive	38	50	2 months; uncomplicated	Slowly progressive dementia last 3 years. Cared for by wife. Diabetes mellitus. Unclassifiable pattern of neural lesions.
Case 11, female S279, consecutive	55	68	6 weeks; uncomplicated	Increasingly forgetful and paranoid since. Cared for by husband. Unclassifiable pattern neural lesions.
Case 12, male S212, consecutive	55	67	4 weeks; uncomplicated	Paranoid delusional psychosis since and dementia. Cared for by wife. Mild brainstem cerebellar syndrome.
Case 13, male S45, consecutive	62	71	3 weeks; uncomplicated	Increasingly poor memory since. Mild hemiparetic pattern of neural lesions.
Case 14, male S67, consecutive	49	66	2 weeks; non-compressive subdural clots	Increasingly forgetful recent years. Mild hemiparetic pattern of neural lesions.
Case 15, female C101, consecutive	51	65	3½ months; internal decompression temporal pole	Increasingly forgetful and having difficulty looking after herself since husband's death 1 year ago. Severe brainstem cerebellar syndrome.
Case 16, male C90, consecutive	53	64	7 months; extradural clot	Increasingly forgetful and ageing prematurely physically since. Mild brainstem cerebellar syndrome.
Case 17, male S167, consecutive	37	47	12 months; uncomplicated	Last 5 years increasing disinhibition, irritability and forgetfulness. Athetoid pseudobulbar pattern.

Table continued overleaf

Table 11.1 – *continued*

Sex and series number	Age at injury	Age examined	Duration PTA and complication	Nature of progressive deterioration and pattern of neural lesions
Case 18, male S59, consecutive	40	56	4 weeks; uncomplicated	Increasingly forgetful and ageing rapidly after initial improvement first 5 years. Brainstem cerebellar syndrome.
Case 19, male S238, consecutive	18	33	10 days; uncomplicated	Increasingly forgetful last five years after initial improvement. Minimal hemiparetic pattern.
Case 20, male A14, selected	25	48	6 months; uncomplicated	Increasingly forgetful and irritable last 3 years. Severe brainstem cerebellar syndrome.
Case 21, female S50, consecutive	12	30	3 weeks; uncomplicated	Demented and childish becoming over the years progressively more irritable and unco-operative. Possibly more a failure to mature as she grew older though also possibly deterioration due to uncontrolled major fits. Mild brainstem cerebellar syndrome.
Case 22, male C9, consecutive	20	33	4 months; acute subdural removal temporal pole, recent second head injury in fit, subdural clot.	Improvement till 8 years after then progressive personality change with ideas influence and reference, and increasing frequency post-traumatic major fits. Probable communicating hydrocephalus following recent second head injury. ?Hypopituitary. Athetoid pseudobulbar syndrome.
Case 23, female C42, consecutive	50	64	Permanent; acute subdural clot	Static after improvement till one of her infrequent post-traumatic fits caused head injury 12 years later and coma half an hour. Progressive dementia and increasing neural disability thereafter suggesting occult hydrocephalus. Static thereafter. Athetoid pseudobulbar with rest tremor one arm.

Case				
Case 24, male A61, selected	22	31	Permanent; acute subdural clot	Poorly controlled post-traumatic epilepsy causing fall 7 years after followed by progressive deterioration in mental and neural disabilities. Confirmed due to external obstructive hydrocephalus. Slow improvement after ventriculo-atrial shunt. Athetoid pseudobulbar.
Case 25, male A8, selected	46	51	Permanent; extradural and subdural clots	Improvement till fall 18 months after then progressively dementing and no longer able to walk as he had. Probable communicating hydrocephalus. Athetoid pseudobulbar syndrome syndrome.
Case 26, male S230, consecutive	36	49	4 weeks; uncomplicated	Increasing spasticity legs last 2 years. Unclassifiable pattern of neural lesions.
Case 27, male C39, consecutive	33	51	3 weeks; acute subdural hygroma	Right hemiparetic limp worse last 5 years. Moderate brainstem cerebellar syndrome.
Case 28, female S280, consecutive	42	52	2½ months; uncomplicated	Improvement then static till 8 years after. Then 'suddenly older', ceased to type with left hand which she had learnt to do, and voice 'quieter'. Athetoid pseudobulbar syndrome.
Case 29, female C26, consecutive	19	37	3 months; acute subdural hygroma	Dense hemiparetic right arm developed clonus on volition 3 years after and not before. Description unlike focal epilepsy or cerebellar tremor and not demonstrable. Severe hemiparetic pattern.
Case 30, female S286, consecutive	40	59	3 months; uncomplicated	Increasingly unsteady walking with more frequent falls last 3 years. Severe brainstem cerebellar syndrome.
Case 31, male A23, selected	23	30	Permanent; uncomplicated	Increasing immobility and slowness of movement last 3 years almost certainly attributable to phenothiazine medication for control of violent rages. Athetoid and parkinsonian pseudobulbar syndrome.

ex-miner at the time of his accident and he continued to drink excessively thereafter until his violent bouts of ill-temper, in which he would assault the brother with whom he lived, finally necessitated his permanent confinement in a psychiatric hospital. Malnutrition due to alcoholism had required a period of hospital care before this, and it seems likely that the combination of alcoholism, serious and permanent brain injury due to the accident and normal ageing accounts for his slowly progressing dementia, of which ill-systematised paranoid delusions were merely one manifestation. These are the only two patients under the age of sixty-five at the time of injury who had suffered a steadily progressing dementia from the time of the injury.

In cases 3–10 in table 11.1 the severity of the intellectual deterioration seems to justify the term 'dementing process'. In all these cases there was a period of improvement after injury, followed by some years during which there was no change in neural function. Then, in each, forgetfulness increased and other manifestations of progressing intellectual and personality decline became evident to the spouse. In cases 3 and 8 this began in their early forties, but in the remainder not for another decade or more. If these are not to be considered due to the effects of ageing on already depleted brain tissue then alternatively the progressing dementias in cases 4, 7 and 9 are indistinguishable from banal senile dementia, and in cases 3, 5, 6 and 8 the intensity of the process and its character suggest the similarly common presenile dementia of Alzheimer although, admittedly, all were deteriorating relatively slowly. In two patients, cases 11 and 12, paranoid delusional symptomatology was the principal manifestation of a progressing mental disorder and although both were evidently forgetful and becoming more so over the years, this was not with the intensity or rapidity usually seen in Alzheimer's disease. It seemed likely that these were both post-traumatic schizophreniform psychoses which were progressing inexorably without treatment. In each case this seemed most likely to reflect severe brain injury compounded by normal ageing.

The next seven patients, cases 13–20, were considered either by themselves or by their spouses or both, to have become increasingly forgetful since their injuries, although this was hardly sufficient to justify the diagnosis of dementia. In half of these patients this became apparent only after a delay of some years, and in the remainder there had been no delay. The severity of the injury in each case varied considerably, as judged by the length of post-traumatic amnesia and the severity and pattern of neural lesions. One patient, case 19, whose injury by these criteria had not been particularly severe, was still relatively young when re-examined, but despite this his increasing forgetfulness seems best explained by the effects of normal ageing superimposed upon traumatic brain damage, as it does also in the other seven patients. The young woman of thirty, case 21, who had become increasingly irritable and difficult to manage as she had grown older, so that she finally had to spend more of her time in a psychiatric hospital than at home, also continued to have uncontrollable generalised convulsions and akinetic attacks. In her case it was most probable that moderately severe traumatic brain damage was being progressively worsened by epileptic hypoxic injury.

In the next four patients, cases 22–25 in table 11.1, a period of improvement after the initial head injury was followed by another more or less severe head injury, all sustained in falls, and thereafter progressive deterioration of both intellectual function and neural disability. In each case the relationship to the second head injury and the clinical picture seemed characteristic of a communicating hydrocephalus of the kind first described by Foltz and Ward (1956) and later in greater detail by Hakim and Adams (1965). In only one case was this diagnosis confirmed by radioisotope cisternography and here marginal improvement occurred with the insertion of a ventriculo-atrial shunt. It was suggested in each of the other cases at the time of re-examination, that a neurosurgical opinion should be sought. In one this diagnosis was entertained but the patient's condition appeared to stabilise and the question of appropriate investigations was postponed whilst she was kept under observation. In another, case 25, the neurosurgeon considered, understandably, that with the development of such a complication in a patient already almost totally incapacitated by the effects of the original injury, further investigation was unwarranted, and the patient progressively deteriorated, dying of bronchopneumonia. The diagnosis remained unconfirmed in case 22, whose second head injury had been complicated by the development of a chronic subdural haematoma. After 6 months there was a gradual spontaneous improvement almost to his former level 10 months after he was seen.

In the remaining six patients the evidence for progression was confined to worsening neural disabilities and did not involve noticeable change in personality or intellect. In case 31 this was apparently attributable to the phenothiazine treatment needed for the patient's otherwise uncontrollable rages. In the remaining five there was no such explanation and the increase in neural disability seemed similar to that seen in ageing cerebral diplegics.

The question of progressive deterioration was further examined by studying the information available from the death certificates of the 206 patients traced from both series who had died, either of the immediate effects of their injury, or subsequently. The details of the causes of death in each case will be referred to in chapter 12. Here mention will be made of those cases in which it seems possible that, although surviving its immediate effects, the injury had nevertheless contributed to premature death. This confines the scrutiny to patients registered as dying from some form of pneumonia. There were four patients who died demented in psychiatric hospitals to which they had been transferred following their injuries. No clear evidence was available in any of these cases to suggest that dementia had actually progressed. All four had, however, died at least two decades before they might reasonably have been expected to actuarially, one in his late forties and the other three in their early fifties. Death occurred 3–8 years after injury.

There were 10 others in the consecutive series of patients, and one in the selected, who were recorded as having died of pneumonia elsewhere than in mental hospitals. Insufficient information was available to show with certainty whether the post-traumatic dementia had progressed in any of these.

All were over the age of fifty-four at the time they were injured. Half died before the age at which death might have been expected in the normal course, suggesting the possibility of the effects of a progressive dementing process. The other half outlived their life expectation to suggest, on the contrary, that there had been no significant progression in their dementias in the years following the injury.

In passing, the question of the frequency with which post-traumatic parkinsonism develops after a single head injury has been answered in the present study. There was not a single case of Parkinson's disease in any of its forms seen among the 331 patients surviving and re-examined, except for the patient already referred to who required high doses of haloperidol. One patient, case 23, had an intermittent rest tremor of her left arm, which neither she nor her husband had noticed. This appeared to have developed after the second head injury, but no other signs were present to justify a diagnosis of Parkinson's disease. On the death certificates of two patients amongst the 206 dead the cause of death included a diagnosis of Parkinson's disease. A prevalence of 1 in 300 cases of Parkinson's disease in patients in their sixties was observed in the community by Brewis, Poskanzer, Rolland and Miller (1966). The occurrence of two cases in the present consecutive series totalling 478 patients is hardly evidence for post-traumatic parkinsonism attributable to a single head injury.

Discussion

The careful study of Corsellis, Bruton and Freeman-Brown (1973) has firmly established that a progressive neuronal degeneration directly attributable to the cumulative effects of repeated head injury of a relatively minor degree, of the kind sustained in boxing, does occasionally occur. Their histological evidence of a hitherto incompletely described and relatively stereotyped constellation of pathological damage, included tears of the septum pellucidum with moderate cerebral atrophy, gliosis and Purkinje cell fallout in the areas of the cerebellar tonsils overlying the foramen magnum, depigmentation of the substantia nigra, atrophy of fornices and mamillary bodies and an unusual distribution of neurofibrillary degeneration. The neuronal degeneration involved the entire cerebral cortex, basal ganglia and diencephalon, but was most intense in the medial temporal grey matter. Typical senile plaques were remarkable for their sparsity or were completely absent. The authors pointed out the striking difference in the distribution of the neuronal degeneration in the brains of these boxers compared with the senile and presenile dementias of Alzheimer, in which the diencephalon and periventricular regions are relatively spared. In the group of unrelated but pathologically similar disorders, which includes the parkinsonian dementia complex of Guam, some forms of chronic encephalitis, Parkinson's disease, especially its post-encephalitic variant and the progressive supranuclear palsy of Steele, Richardson and Olszewski (1964), the cerebral hemispheres are relatively spared and the brunt of the neurofibrillary degeneration falls on the neurones in the mid-brain, pons and medulla. These authors considered that the evidence they had presented strongly suggested that the repeated cerebral traumata of boxing should be added to the list of precipitating, if not causal, agents of neurofibrillary degeneration, and that, in the absence of senile plaques, the effects of ageing could not be held responsible.

Evidence that any similar process may be precipitated by a single injury to the head, however severe, is still lacking. The belief that it does is supported by anecdotal reference to the occasional case in which a progressive dementing process has followed a single head injury. This has been noted by, amongst others, Bowman and Blau (1960), Claude and Cuel (1939) and Corsellis and Brierley (1959). These latter authors were at pains to point out the possibility that the head injury and subsequent dementia were coincidentally rather than causally related, and drew attention to the need to follow all such cases 'through to the end', so that, even if the underlying pathological changes only rarely turned out to be those of a progressive neuronal degeneration, it would be of interest to establish what these were. In an unpublished thesis Hollander (1968), and later Hollander and Strich (1970), described the case of a woman aged sixty-six who fell downstairs, subsequently had the resulting subdural hygromas drained and then recovered from the immediate effects of her injury, only to become progressively and profoundly demented in the course of the next 3 years. The histological changes they found in her brain were those of Alzheimer's disease together with congophilic angiopathy. In the same paper the authors reported two similar cases following subarachnoid haemorrhage, and discussed the possibility that trauma and the insult produced by subarachnoid bleeding might have been responsible for the pathological process they found. In the case described by Corsellis and Brierley (1959) and one of those of Hollander and Strich (1970) there were parkinsonian features of rigidity and tremor associated with the dementia.

In the present study the most careful enquiry for the slightest evidence of progressive neurological disease after a single major head injury has produced amongst the survivors only the 31 cases tabulated above. Analysis of the form this deterioration had taken in the individual case, the speed of its development, the delay after the injury, the age of the patient, the severity of the injury as judged by the length of the post-traumatic amnesia, the pattern of neural lesions, and the associated factors of epilepsy and alcoholism, does not provide striking evidence of a specific neuronal degeneration due to a single head injury. Nor, in a review of the cause of death amongst the remaining patients no longer alive at the time of the follow-up study, was there any convincing evidence to support such a concept.

The evidence required in a study of this kind which would have supported the entity of progressive traumatic encephalopathy provoked by a single head injury, should have shown, as in the progressive encephalopathy of boxers, that there was some relation between the type and severity of the head injury, and perhaps also some discernible pattern of neural lesions. On the contrary, in the above tabulation it may be seen that such correlations were significantly absent, and it was notable that there were six patients whose neural lesions were not classifiable in terms of the four patterns most commonly observed in the study. In other words, amongst the patients who deteriorated progressively after their injuries there were 20 per cent whose neural lesions could not be classified, compared with 10 per cent in the entire consecutive series.

On the other hand, although among the 37 'punch-drunk' ex-professional boxers examined by Roberts (1969) the author accepted four cases as having progressively deteriorated in a manner that was unlikely to be attributable to normal ageing, there was no good evidence among the rest that a specific neuronal degeneration rather than age was the cause. In the light of the more recent pathological evidence produced by Corsellis, Bruton and Freeman-Browne (1973), it seems possible that the brains of at least some of those who had exhibited late and progressive deterioration, which had seemed likely to be due to ageing, might have had the extensive neurofibrillary degenerative process without plaques described by these authors.

In the absence of pathological data for those patients in the present study who did progressively deteriorate, the most probable explanation for their deterioration is that ageing was superimposed upon a brain, the 'functional reserve' of which had already been severely depleted by the injury. This concept of a single head injury depleting the neuronal functional reserve seems first to have been suggested by Symonds (1937) and later expanded (Symonds, 1962) to explain his own observation that a second head injury may produce permanent intellectual impairment and personality disorder, out of all proportion to the severity of the injury judged by the duration of the post-traumatic amnesia.

The specific effects of ageing on an already damaged brain were examined by Ciompi (1972) and in a more detailed study of the same series of patients by Daghighian (1973). These authors followed a series of patients treated in a psychiatric hospital after head injury sustained at an average of fifty-one years. There were 26 survivors and their average age was seventy-two at the time of re-examination. Comparing the ageing of their patients with those amongst the psychiatric community who had not had head injuries, the authors concluded that evidence of organic deterioration at an advanced age was probably more frequent amongst the patients who had sustained head injuries. Ortegasuhrkamp, Faust and Schulte (1975) also found premature ageing in a substantial proportion of patients who had sustained head injuries when they were middle-aged and elderly. In neither of these studies was it the particular concern of the authors to estimate the prevalence of progressive dementia in an unselected population of the severely injured, but their findings do seem relevant and provide some support for the contention that it is the effects of ageing on a brain already depleted of a substantial proportion of neurones, which explains most cases of progressing dementia after head injury. The only patients in the present study whose late deterioration was characteristic of the neurological syndrome of occult communicating hydrocephalus had all developed it after further head injuries. Although a relatively frequent sequel of severe head injury in the short-term, according to, amongst others, Pedersen and Haase (1973), Granholm and Svendgaard (1972), Salmon and Timperman (1971) and Lewin (1968a), there is no good evidence to indicate how often it is a complication developing only many years later without the provocation of another head injury. On the evidence of the present study it would seem to be an extremely rare event.

It is hardly conceivable that, if there were such an entity as a specific neuronal degeneration induced by a single head injury and occurring with the frequency of the progressing post-traumatic dementias observed in this study, its pathology would have been overlooked until now. According to Logan and Cushion (1958), and Brewis, Poskanzer, Rolland and Miller (1966) there are no figures available to indicate the prevalence of dementia in the community, nor, according to Corsellis (1962, 1976) of Alzheimer's presenile dementia, due to overdiagnosis of cerebrovascular disease. In a study of the prevalence of dementia among those aged 65 and older in the general population Kay, Beamish and Roth (1964) found about 5 per cent dementing due to varying degrees of a 'senile brain syndrome'. In the present study there were 9 of 72 patients, that is 12 per cent, of this age progressively dementing from what would seem to be a comparable disorder among the consecutive series. These can be identified in table 11.1, excluding the two patients, cases 13 and 14, with only increasing forgetfulness. Estimates of the large numbers of patients in the community who survive a head injury which causes post-traumatic amnesia of a week or longer, are made in chapter 13. Suffice it to note here that a slowly progressing dementia following a severe head injury, either from the time of the injury, or after a delay of a few years, far from being a rarity, is a relatively common occurrence. As a corollary to this the question which remains to be answered is whether a single severe head injury may actually accelerate the process of normal brain ageing, or precipitate or enhance the senile and presenile degenerative changes of Alzheimer's disease. On this point the data derived from the present study suggest that it may do both, but pathological confirmation is lacking.

12 Life Expectancy and Causes of Death

The majority who survived their injury in coma or post-traumatic amnesia for a week and then succumbed before recovering sufficiently to be discharged from hospital, died in the first 3 months after injury. In table 12.1 the period

Table 12.1   Deaths due to the 'immediate'* effects of the head injury and period of survival

	Age at injury			
	5–25	26–45	46–55	56+
Number of consecutive series patients surviving				
1 week+ to 3 months	16	15	11	48
3 months+ to 1 year	1	3		6
1 year+	1	2		
Totals	18	20	11	54
Number of selected series patients surviving †				
1 to 3 months	7	7	3	14
3 months to 1 year	8	10		6
1 year+	6	2	2	1
Totals	21	19	5	21

Consecutive series, total 103 patients; selected series, total 66 patients.
* 'Immediate': This includes all patients dying however long after their head injury whose recovery was never sufficient to enable them to leave hospital. Most remained apallic, unconscious or delirious till death. The causes of death of all patients not included above are given in table 12.2.
† Comprises 43 Army and Addenbrooke's with 43 consecutive.

of survival and the age at which the patient was injured are set out for both the consecutive and selected series. Although survival was in some cases remarkably protracted, in these patients death has been attributed to the 'immediate' effects of the injury in order to distinguish between life expectancy in patients who 'recover' from their injuries and leave hospital, and in those who do not. The majority of deaths are recorded in death certificates and hospital notes as being due to head injury, with or without mention of associated pneumonia and other systemic complications of inanition and decubitus. Most remained unconscious or demented until they died.

Extracting from these cases all who remained in various states of tonic decerebration and altered consciousness until death, it may again be seen, in figure 12.1, that most were dead within the year but that there were some very long survivals. Included amongst these are patients who remained completely mute and akinetic except for reflex extension or flexion in response to stimulation, and also those who, after surviving in this state for various

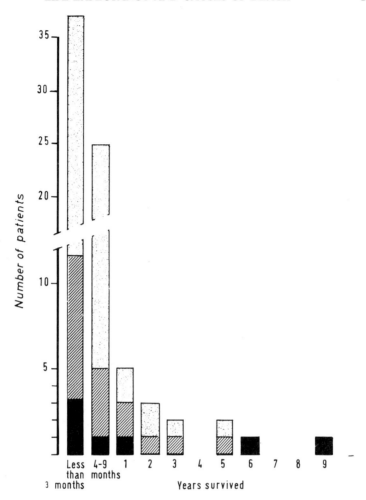

Figure 12.1   Survival after severe head injury in states of 'dementia and decerebration', N=76 patients. Ages of patients at injury are indicated as follows:
▨, 26+ years; ▨, 16–25 years; ■, 5–15 years.

periods, finally developed some form of semi-purposive or near-purposive
movement, usually in a single limb. These patients often recovered a level of
neural responsiveness that permitted the expression of primitive emotions of
pleasure, pain and anger, and there was the occasional patient who could utter
a poorly articulated word or two. The justification for including all these cases
in one group, despite very obvious differences between total mute akinesia in
deep coma, or 'coma vigil' and those patients who, whilst still in tonic
decerebration and profoundly demented, may display emotion and some
form of movement or sound indicative of a higher level of neural integration,
has been the natural history of the condition observed in the present study.
This is in striking contrast to the relatively normal life expectancy of most

patients with the two syndromes designated athetoid pseudobulbar and brainstem cerebellar. In the present study there was no case surviving decerebrate in coma for longer than 3 months whose condition altered materially thereafter so that it could be reclassified as athetoid pseudobulbar or brainstem cerebellar. In other words, it seemed that although there was the possibility of some marginal increase in the range of emotional response and movement, where the syndrome of decerebrate dementia had persisted unchanged for 3 months it was thereafter permanent until death, reflecting profound and irrecoverable neural damage. There has been no patient examined for the purposes of this study who has yet survived in this state for longer than 10 years.

Turning now to those patients in the consecutive series who survived the 'immediate' effects of their injuries and recovered sufficiently to return to the community, table 12.2 records the cause of death of each patient found to have died at some time between leaving hospital and the follow-up study 10–24 years later.

Life expectancy, or more accurately, the risk of death among these patients in the first 20 years after their head injury, is shown graphically in figure 12.2 compared with the life expectancy for each age group amongst the general

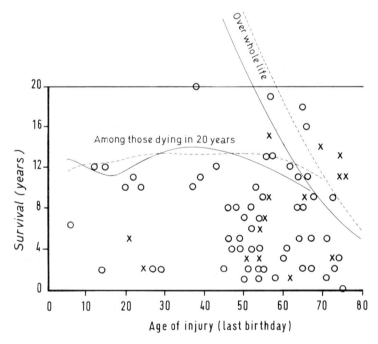

Figure 12.2   Survival period in years plotted against age at injury for those 75 individuals from the consecutive series who died after surviving the 'immediate' effects of the closed head injury sufficiently 'recovered' to leave hospital. O, Males; ×, females; ——, life table expectation for males; – – – –, life table expectation for females.

Table 12.2   Cause of death, age at injury and death of survivors of 'immediate' effects of head injury

	Age at injury	Age at death	Cause of death	PTA (weeks)
Age at injury 5–15 (life expectancy 70 years)				
48 examined	12	24	Disseminated sclerosis	2
	5	11	Epilepsy, during serial fits*	24+
3 dead 'immediate' effect	14	16	Drowning, accidental	24+
4 dead, survived 'immediate' effects	15	27	Another traffic accident, motor-cycle	6
Age at injury 16–25 (life expectancy 70 years)				
101 examined	20	30	Electrocuted, accident at work	1½
	21 F	26	Suicide by gas*	12
15 dead 'immediate' effects	22	33	Epilepsy, in a fit*	5
5 dead, survived 'immediate' effects	24	34	Tuberculous meningitis	3
	25 F	27	Pneumococcal meningitis*	16
Age at injury 26–35 (life expectancy 71 years)				
52 examined	27	29	Drowning, accidental	6
	29	31	Another racing motor-cycle accident	4
11 dead 'immediate' effects				
2 dead, survived 'immediate' effects				
Age at injury 36–45 (life expectancy 71 years)				
40 examined	37	47	Drowning, accidental	4
	38	58	Cor pulmonale, chronic bronchitis	3
9 dead 'immediate' effects	39	50	Epilepsy, in status*	6
5 dead, survived 'immediate' effects	43	55	Stroke	24+
	45	47	Bronchopneumonia	24+

Table 12.2 continued overleaf

Table 12.2 — continued

Age at injury	Age at death	Cause of death	PTA (weeks)
Age at injury 46–55 (life expectancy 72–3 years)			
36 examined			
11 dead 'immediate' effects			
23 dead, survived 'immediate' effects			
46	51	Coronary	24
46	54	Bronchopneumonia	24+
47	51	Accident at work on railway	4
48	56	Coronary	4
48	52	Coronary	3
49	54	Coronary	4
50	51	Coronary	5
50	57	Malignant cerebral glioma	24
51	53	Stroke	20
51 F	54	Bronchopneumonia	24+
52	58	Coronary	8
52	60	Carcinoma stomach	4
52	56	Pneumococcal meningitis*	3
53	63	Coronary	1
54	55	Suicide by aspirin*	24+
54 F	57	Bronchopneumonia	3
54	64	Coronary	3
54	61	Stroke	1
54	56	Carcinoma lung	5
54 F	59	Bronchopneumonia	24+
55	64	Carcinoma stomach	2
55	57	Carcinomatosis	3
55 F	62	Another traffic accident	2
Age at injury 56–65 (life expectancy 73–7 years)			
13 examined			
21 dead 'immediate' effects			
17 dead, survived 'immediate' effects			
56 F	65	Hypertensive cardiac failure	1
56	69	Another accidental head injury in fall	3
57	76	Coronary	6
57 F	72	Carcinoma bladder	4
57	70	Suicide by barbiturates	3

Age at injury	Cause of death	
58	Carcinomatosis	1
60	Carcinoma lung	2
61	Bronchopneumonia	24+
62 F	Pneumococcal meningitis*	1½
62	Cardiac failure	2
63 F	Bronchopneumonia	4
64	Bronchopneumonia	24+
64	Carcinoma colon	8
64	Coronary	5
65	Bronchopneumonia	24+
65	Stroke	3
65	Stroke	2
66	Stroke, Parkinson's disease	4
66 F	Carcinoma breast	4
66	Bronchopneumonia	24
67	Cor pulmonale, chronic bronchitis	2
67	Uraemia	2
67	Bronchopneumonia	12
68	Bronchopneumonia	24
71	Bronchopneumonia	24+
70 F	Bronchopneumonia	3
71	Another accidental head injury and fall	4
71	Epilepsy causing fall, head injury and death after venous thrombosis and pulmonary embolus*	3
73 F	Carcinoma stomach	6
73	Coronary	6
73	Stroke	24+
74	Bronchopneumonia	24+
75 F	Coronary	2
75 F	Stroke, Parkinson's disease	3
75	Cardiac failure	2
77 F	Coronary	24+

Age at injury 66–77 (life expectancy 77–83 years)
Age at injury 78–85 (life expectancy 84–89 years)
1 examined
24 dead 'immediate' effects
19 dead, survived 'immediate' effects

Consecutive series, total 469 patients: 291 examined; 103 dead of 'immediate' effects; 75 dead, survived 'immediate' effects.
* Death unquestionably causally related to head injury.

population. The English Life Tables for the year 1960 (1962) have been used as they seemed the most appropriate to the period under review. The median survival in years for each age group, compared with the general population, and the median shortfall are given in table 12.3. It may be seen from table

Table 12.3　Median survival (years) among those who died (consecutive series), compared with a median survival of 12 years* among those dying within 20 years, in the general population

Age	Median survival	Shortfall over median in general population
16–35	5	7
36–45	11	1
46–55	5	7
56–65	9	3
66+	9	3
Average		5

* From English Life Table (1960).

12.4 that the chances of death occurring in the first 20 years after injury are no greater, except in children, than in the general population, but from table 12.3 that the life expectancy of those who have sustained a head injury of this severity appears to be reduced on average by about 5 years. It might be assumed that this reduction in life expectancy extends beyond the 24 years after head injury covered by the follow-up period in this study.

Table 12.4　Statistical significance of tests of two null hypotheses*

Age range	Number surviving 'immediate' effects	Number dead within 20 years			Of those dead in 20 years, number dead before or after conditional median age death		
		Observed	Expected	Sig.	Before	After	Sig.
5–15	52	4	0.89	$P=0.012$	2	2	Not sig.
16–25	106	5	2.76	Not sig.	5	0	$P<0.001$
26–35	54	2	2.94	Not sig.	2	0	
36–45	45	5	7.13	Not sig.	4	1	
46–55	59	23	23.1	Not sig.	23	0	
56–65	30	17	21.3	Not sig.	9	8	Not sig.
66+	20	19	19.71	Not sig.	9	10	Not sig.

All statistical significance tests are 'one tail'. They are chi-squared or exact binomial tests, as appropriate.
* The two null hypotheses are as follows:
　I　That the proportion dead within 20 years does not differ between the group with head injuries, and the general population.
　II　That the probability of surviving beyond the median age of death is 50 per cent among those who die within 20 years.

An examination of the causes of death in the individual cases, however, raises doubts as to whether such overall estimates of the reduction in life expectancy are justifiable. These suggest that, instead of death from natural causes being accelerated in some inexplicable manner by the head injury, a more accurate method of interpreting the information would be to consider specifically those factors likely to reduce life expectancy in each case, accepting that where these are not present, life expectation is unaltered. It is difficult, for example, to see how carcinoma of the bronchus, breast, stomach or colon can be attributable in any way to the head injury, or, for that matter, how premature death from myocardial or cerebral infarction or hypertensive cardiac failure, many years after a head injury, could be related to this at all. Even accepting the view that stress or lack of exercise contributes to the development of atheromatous arterial disease, it does not seem very likely that a head injury sustained by a man in his thirties or forties will add much to the already considerable risk run by men in the general population of developing and finally succumbing to the various manifestations of atherosclerosis. A comparison of the proportions of the population dying from these serious conditions, derived from the *Registrar General's Statistical Review of England and Wales 1960* (1962) is given in table 12.5. This does not suggest that there is any increased incidence amongst the head-injured patients.

Table 12.5   Deaths from selected causes among the 75 severely head injured patients of the consecutive series who survived the 'immediate' effects of their injuries compared with proportionate numbers dying from similar causes derived from the death rates reported in the *Registrar General's Statistical Review of England and Wales 1960*

Cause of death	Deaths among severely head injured	Deaths among population of England and Wales	Increased risk of death after severe head injury	Sig.
Meningitis	4	0.06	×65	$P<0.001$
Epilepsy	4	0.1	×40	$P<0.001$
Drowning	3	0.15	×20	$P<0.001$
Accidents	7	2	×3	Not sig.
Suicide	3	1	×3	Not sig.
Respiratory disease	17	8	×2	$P<0.005$
Cardiovascular disease	16	16	The same	
Malignant disease	11	14	Slightly less	
Cerebrovascular disease	8	10	Slightly less	

The immediate relevance of the head injury to premature death from post-traumatic epilepsy and meningitis is unquestionable, however. It is also clear that suicide and accidental death by drowning has occurred with greater frequency here than in the general population. However, even in these patients a closer look at the individual cases must result in the exclusion of one patient who died of tuberculous meningitis, and raise doubts about the relevance of the head injury in the case of the patient who committed suicide where it was noted on the death certificate that he also had carcinoma of the lip. There is insufficient information available to decide in retrospect whether the latter contributed in any way to the man's decision to kill himself or was merely an incidental finding at the coroner's post-mortem.

The extent to which the head injury may be held to have contributed to premature death, when this was recorded as due to pneumonia, has been examined briefly in the preceding chapter. It would seem that where post-traumatic dementia is severe enough to necessitate permanent care in a mental hospital, the head injury is directly implicated in premature death from bronchopneumonia. This also seems to be the case when dementia has necessitated admission to a geriatric unit. Premature death occurred in three out of four patients who died demented in a geriatric hospital, but it should be noted that one survived there longer than would have been actuarially expected.

There is surprisingly little evidence to implicate with certainty other post-traumatic mental or physical disabilities as a cause of early death in those who survived the immediate effects of their head injury. Of the three cases of drowning only two had severe physical disability, but impaired vestibular function may well have been present in all. Only one of the three patients who committed suicide had severe physical disability. The dementia which necessitated permanent institutional care in mental hospitals was clearly highly relevant to the premature deaths of three patients, and this is probably also true of most of the 10 remaining demented patients who died of bronchopneumonia. In the case of the three patients who died as a result of further road traffic accidents it is clear that only one had serious residual physical disability and some frontal personality change. One of the other two patients was well enough to kill himself in another motor-cycle race, whilst the other had returned to riding his motor-cycle normally on the roads. Since in both these cases the first and second accidents were virtually identical, there are no grounds for suggesting that a frontal personality change due to the first injury was the cause of the second, rather than a constitutional proneness to accidents. Again it is doubtful what contribution traumatic personality change might have made in the case of death from electrocution at work. No clear relationship is apparent between the severity of the head injury, as judged by the length of post-traumatic amnesia, and premature death, amongst those who survived the immediate effects of their injuries, except in the case of those whose deaths were recorded as due to pneumonia.

Discussion

There are serious limitations to any attempt at generalisation about life expectancy on the basis of a small number of patients. A small series does, however, allow a more detailed analysis of the cause of death in each case and a more realistic assessment of its relevance to the head injury. To improve on estimates of life expectancy derived from studies of small numbers of men followed by Walker and Erculei (1969) for over 15 years after their war injuries, Walker, Leuchs, Lechtape-Grüter, Caveness, and Kretschman (1971) studied ex-soldiers injured in the First World War. The records of these cases were in the archives of the Hirnverletzternheim in Munich. The hospital had been established for the treatment of the brain-injured in 1916 and later became the head injury centre for the Bavarian army, all soldiers from the region who had survived their head injuries being sent there for assessment of disability and compensation. From the total of 5500 records of head-injured patients, which included field medical and sequential neurological reports, a random selection was made of 1000 case records from amongst those containing sufficient information for an analysis of the type of injury, the initial and late neurological states, and the subsequent medical social and economic progress. The dates and causes of death were established from this and other sources for approximately 600 of these cases. For a variety of reasons the remainder were untraced. A control series of unwounded Bavarian veterans of the First World War who had been decorated and received pensions was compiled from the files of the Social Welfare Department. A comparable series of 600 patients, for whom the cause of death could be established, was selected from amongst these. The head injuries were a mixed series of both penetrating missile and closed injuries. All degrees of severity were included, even just scalp lacerations. Life expectancy tables were constructed for the control and wounded soldiers. It was found, for both epileptic and non-epileptic patients, that those who had sustained a head injury had a life expectancy which was about 4 years shorter at all ages than that of the control group. There was little evidence to suggest that post-traumatic epilepsy itself made any substantial contribution to premature death, since few men had actually died during a fit. In general the causes of death in the head-injured were similar, both qualitatively and quantitatively, to those in the general population. The authors speculate that since life expectancy was less for both epileptic and non-epilectic head-injured men the important factor determining the reduction in life expectancy was probably brain damage. It seemed to them that the cumulative effects of traumatic brain damage and ageing might reduce the ability of the brain to compensate with age, although whether this was because of 'vascular or neuronal deficiency' was unclear. They proposed that subtle functional changes induced by various 'cerebral impairments resulting from head injury rendered the general defence mechanisms of the body more vulnerable to the stresses of ageing'. This seems to be a statement in other words of Symonds' (1962) concept of the limited 'functional reserve' of the brain which may be revealed by the effects of a second head injury on a previously injured brain. The more detailed analysis of the information available in the present study on the causes of death and their relationship to the severity of the injury provides some minimal support for this idea, but only in the case of those few patients who died prematurely with dementia or bronchopneumonia. The evidence presented here does not suggest that coronary or cerebral atheroma or cerebral or systemic neoplastic disease has been hastened or caused by the severe head injuries these patients sustained. It is more likely that the overall reduction in life expectancy of 4–5 years estimated on the basis of the data derived from the present study is to be accounted for by certain specific factors which in individual cases have increased the risks of death from pneumococcal meningitis, epilepsy, suicide, accidents, notably drowning, and respiratory disease. In table 12.5 it was seen that only when due to these causes has death exceeded, proportionately, the numbers occurring in the general population.

As to life expectancy and the causes of death amongst those who died of the immediate effects of their head injury, however long afterwards, the data derived from the present study bear comparison with those presented by Carlsson, Essen and Löfgren (1968). In their examination of the factors affecting mortality after head injury these authors studied the case records of 496 patients admitted to a neurosurgical unit after closed head injury over a 10-year period. Only those patients who died from their injury without having regained consciousness, or who survived after a post-traumatic coma of more than 12 hours' duration were selected for study. Unconsciousness was assumed to have persisted until the patient responded verbally, however inadequately, to the spoken word. Complicated injuries requiring neurosurgical treatment were excluded, amongst them patients with brain lacerations and brain swelling associated with cerebral contusion. The overall mortality was 34 per cent. The authors felt that in 28 per cent of these the probable cause of death was primary cerebral injury, in 6 per cent various extracranial complications, and in the remaining two-thirds pneumonia, thromboembolism, gastrointestinal haemorrhage, myocardial infarction, uraemia and meningitis. They drew attention to the fact that these latter complications of head injury occurred almost exclusively and increasingly in the higher age groups.

The period of survival was very different amongst those whose death was considered to be due to primary brain damage, where 96 per cent were dead within 48 hours of the injury. Deaths due to secondary causes occurred most frequently between the fourth and 22nd day, the majority during the second week. The authors show that this tendency to die of the primary effects of the brain trauma is unrelated to the age of the patient except for those under the age of ten at the time of injury. It may be assumed, they conclude, that the injury has not been of a severity to cause lethal brain damage if, after the establishment of a free airway, there is some improvement in the clinical state of the patient. Death is then due not to the trauma itself but to systemic complications which increase in frequency with age. Only five of their patients who survived their injuries for 48 hours then failed to regain consciousness so that verbal contact could be established. The state of these patients underwent a gradual change from decerebration and deep coma to a condition typical of the apallic syndrome. In their series the longest period of coma which was consistent with a recovery of consciousness was 13 weeks. These authors do not discuss the frequency with which cerebral perfusion failure, hypoxia and brain swelling, rather than the mechanical effects of the trauma, were responsible for death in those held to have died from lethal brain injury rather than secondary systemic effects.

The present study is heavily biased towards more severe brain injury. The distinction between death due to primary traumatic damage, either mechanical or due to perfusion failure and hypoxia, and that due to secondary systemic effects, seems nevertheless to be supported. It is clear, however, that in most patients with the syndrome of decerebrate dementia recorded as dying of bronchopneumonia, the severity of the injury itself can hardly have been compatible with other than more or less limited survival. There is little published information on the question of life expectancy in states of decerebrate dementia. Vigouraux, Baurand, Choux and Guillermain (1972) report on an apallic patient who survived for 11 years and Ingvar (1975) refers briefly to one patient surviving in this state for 15 years. Gammie (1977) recently observed survival in this state for 18 years of a man injured in his early forties. The possibility of 'indefinite' survival in these 'vegetative' states has been mentioned by Jennett and Plum (1972), and by Vapalahti and Troupp (1971), but these authors do not provide any evidence that this does occur nor numerical data as to the most probable period of survival in this state after head injury. The information presented in this study suggests that these forms of 'posthumous' existence, as Vapalahti and Troupp have aptly described them, will very rarely be prolonged more than 10 years after injury.

13 Predicting the Long-term Outcome

Brief reference to this aspect of the assessment of the long-term outcome has already been made both in the review of previous reports and, in passing, in several earlier chapters. The relationship is examined here between a number of features of the acute and convalescent periods after injury, including the various indirect measures of severity already defined, which seem likely indices of the outcome observed 10–25 years later. Their reliability as predictors in the long-term is then assessed. The data have been studied in three ways. In the first a graphic method has been used to examine selected information available for only the majority of the cases; in the second a computer-assisted numerical analysis has been made; and in the third 'flow diagrams' have been drawn to summarise the prediction procedure implied by the statistical analysis.

Graphic Method

The central neural disability grading scale defined in table 5.1 on page 40 and a semi-logarithmic time-scale were used to construct graphs to examine the time course of recovery for patients injured at different ages. In figures 13.1 (a), (b) and 13.2(a) the recovery curves for patients from the consecutive series with uncomplicated injuries and coma lasting less than a month who were left with no central neural disability are compared with the recovery curves of patients who were left with a degree of central neural disability graded slight or worse. Points were plotted, white for those left with no disability and black for those left with disability graded slight or worse, in the case of every patient for whom there was information in the hospital records at selected time intervals during the acute and convalescent periods after injury. Thereafter the information plotted was taken from the patients themselves and their relatives at the time they were reviewed. Understandably more data were recorded in the hospital notes, and at more frequent intervals for patients whose injuries were severe or complicated, and whose convalescence was protracted, than for those whose recovery was rapid.

It was also clear from these graphs that the rate of recovery is closely related to the long-term outcome. Whether in the acute stage after injury there was decerebration, or purposive and semi-purposive movement in response to stimulation, or merely bedbound confusion, also indicates the likely long-term prognosis, but there is overlap between these indices and outcome, and it appears from the graphs that the rate of recovery more clearly predicts outcome than does the worst state of neurological responsiveness recorded in hospital after injury.

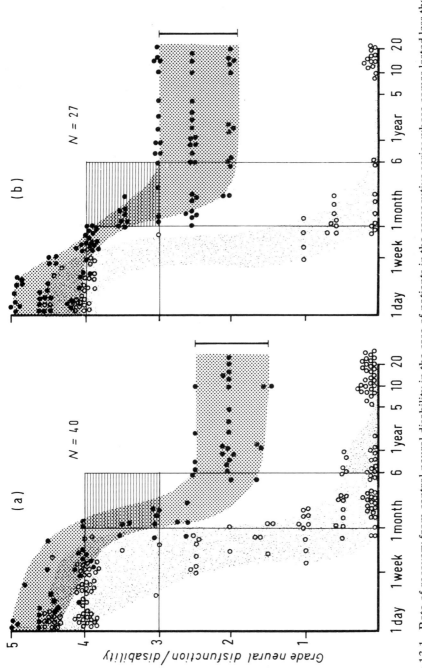

Figure 13.1 Rate of recovery from central neural disability in the case of patients in the consecutive series whose comas lasted less than 1 month. (a) Patients with uncomplicated injuries injured between the ages of sixteen and twenty-five; (b) patients with uncomplicated injuries injured between the ages of twenty-six and forty-five.

The grades of neural dysfunction/disability are as follows: 5, decerebrate; 4, bedbound; 3, severe disability but walking unassisted; 2, moderate disability; 1, slight disability. ○, Patients who ultimately had no neurophysical disability; ●, patients who ultimately had a disability graded as slight or worse.

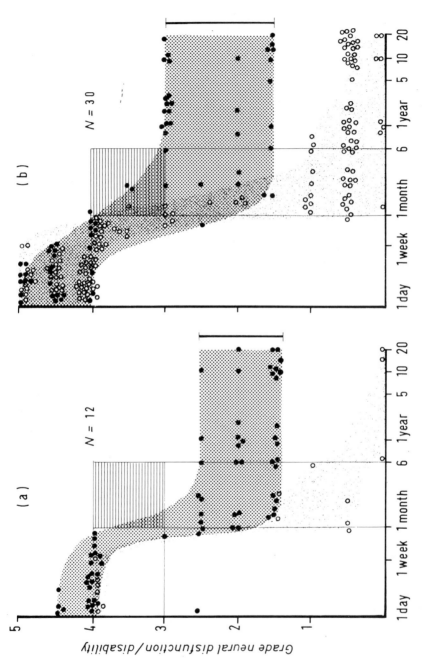

Figure 13.2   Rate of recovery from central nervous disability in the case of patients in the consecutive series whose comas lasted for less than 1 month. (a) Patients injured at the age of fifty-five or more with uncomplicated injuries; (b) patients injured between the ages of sixteen and forty-five with complicated injuries. For legend see caption to figure 13.1.

Comparing the three age groups it is also apparent that amongst those who were injured between the ages of sixteen and twenty-five, whose injuries were uncomplicated and caused coma lasting less than a month, very few were left with any disability at all. Amongst those who were 10–25 years older at the time of injury fewer made a complete recovery and many were left with more severe grades of disability. Among those older than forty-five when they were injured none initially decerebrate survived to be followed up, but of those who were not decerebrate and who did survive to be reviewed only one was severely disabled by central neural lesions.

No one walking unassisted within 3 weeks of injury, and very few walking unassisted within a month, had any central neural disability in the long-term.

The time course of recovery in injury complicated by extradural or subdural haematoma or brain penetration, whether this was traumatic or surgical (the latter, as has already been described, usually undertaken for internal decompression of lacerated brain with or without associated intra- or extracerebral bleeding) is illustrated in figure 13.2(b). In many patients who became decerebrate for only short periods before operation ultimate disability was minimal, clearly indicating that the concussive brain injury was not severe, and that secondary infarction due to compression was avoided by the decompressive procedure. On the other hand, varying degrees of cerebral infarction due to prolonged compression are likely to account for the fact that more in each age group amongst these patients with complicated injuries are left with more severe grades of disability than is the case amongst those whose injuries were uncomplicated. The time scale of recovery is lengthened, but again it is the rate at which this takes place which seems most closely related to the final degree of disability.

Combining two groups of patients injured between the ages of sixteen and twenty-five, and twenty-six and forty-five years whose residual disability was negligible or minimal it may be seen in figure 13.3(a) that rapid improvement in the first month accurately predicts the ultimate outcome, though there may be moderate disability persisting for as long as 18 months.

In figure 13.4(a) and (b) individual recovery curves have been drawn for each patient with an uncomplicated injury which had caused unconsciousness prolonged for a month or more. The striking feature of these injuries, judged more severe solely by the indirect measure of the duration of coma, is the contrast between the two age groups. Children injured between the ages of five and fifteen, even though decerebrate for a week and unconscious for a month or longer, and hardly walking without assistance by a year, continued to improve slowly over many years and the final degree of central neural disability was often mild, or at least no more than moderately incapacitating in domestic, social or occupational spheres of activity. Indeed it appeared that decerebration for longer than $2\frac{1}{2}$ weeks in children was compatible with little neurophysical disability in the long-term. It is therefore clear that the degree of initial central neural dysfunction overestimates the extent of irreversible brain damage in children. In contrast, decerebration in adults of more than $2\frac{1}{2}$

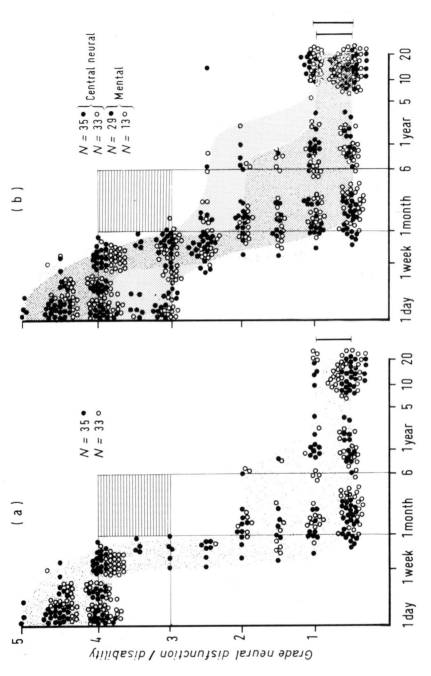

Figure 13.3 Rate of recovery of patients from the consecutive series who had a disability graded as minimal or negligible and whose comas lasted less than 1 month. (a) Central neural disability; (b) mental disability superimposed on the central neural disability shown in (a). ●, Patients with uncomplicated injuries aged between sixteen and twenty-five at injury; ○, patients with uncomplicated injuries aged between twenty-six and forty-five at injury.

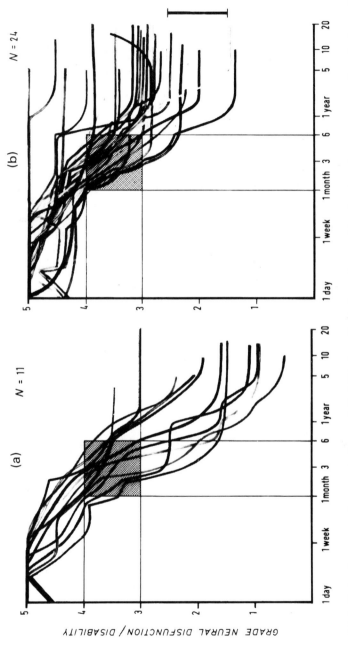

Figure 13.4 Rate of recovery from central neural disability in patients from the combined series who were unconscious for 1 month or more with an uncomplicated injury. (a) Patients aged between five and fifteen at injury; (b) patients of sixteen or more years of age at injury.

weeks duration invariably resulted in severe and permanent neurophysical disability, precluding a normal social, domestic and occupational life, though in a number of cases the degree of disability was not enough to prevent unassisted walking eventually. No patient decerebrate for longer than 3 months in this series ever recovered beyond a vegetative or analogous state. Furthermore, when in adults coma had lasted longer than a month, and then walking unassisted was delayed longer than 3 months, there was always profound persisting neurophysical disability precluding normal domestic, social or occupational life. In contrast, amongst adults walking unassisted within 3 months the likelihood of there being more than moderate to severe neurophysical disability in the long-term was slight.

In figure 13.3(b) a comparison has been made between the rate of recovery of disability due to central neural lesions and the rate of recovery of disability due to intellectual impairment or personality change. This has been done by superimposing a graph of the mental disability recovery curve for the same patients whose central neural recovery is illustrated in figure 13.3(a). Recovery from neurophysical disability is evidently in general more rapid than recovery from mental disability. These graphs also show that with increasing age there are more patients left with those minimal degrees of central neural disability than with no disability at all, or with degrees of disability graded moderate or worse. Of those aged sixteen to twenty-five (35 out of 81) at injury 43 per cent were left with this minimal degree of central neural disability compared with 53 per cent (33 out of 62) of those who were 10–20 years older. The situation is reversed with mental disability. Fewer, that is 21 per cent (13 out of 62), among those aged between twenty-six and forty-five are left with the minimal degrees of mental disability rather than no disability or severer grades, compared with 36 per cent (29 out of 81) of those injured when 10–20 years younger.

These graphic illustrations of the time course of recovery obscure the observation repeatedly made in this study of almost indefinite continuing improvement which may be seen in both mental and central neural traumatic sequelae. This was particularly striking in the case of children injured before the age of fifteen, but it was even apparent in two adolescents with decerebrate dementia. Akinetic mutism for 3 years did not preclude the recovery of limited monosyllabic speech in two cases. The period over which recovery could be expected to continue and its tempo were closely related to age, as well as to the severity and nature of the disabilities.

The time course of recovery in the case of two groups of patients injured between the ages of sixteen and twenty-five, and twenty-six and forty-five, who were left with mental disability graded slight or worse is illustrated in figure 13.5. The slower rate of recovery from intellectual impairment and personality disorder is apparent, as also is the larger number left with substantial mental disability in this same group of adults whose neurophysical rate of recovery has already been illustrated in figure 13.1(a) and (b).

Implicit in accepting that the rate of recovery, as shown in these graphs,

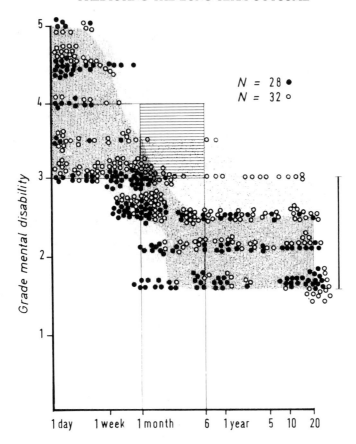

Figure 13.5   Rate of recovery from mental disability of patients from the consecutive
series with uncomplicated injuries who had been in a coma for less than 1
month and who had ultimately a mental disability graded as slight or
worse. ●, Patients injured between the ages of sixteen and twenty-five;
O, patients injured between the ages of twenty-six and forty-five.

does have predictive value in the long-term, is the assumption that, had
recorded data in the hospital notes been uniformly available at each of the
selected intervals of time after injury for the entire population studied, they
would not have differed materially from those available in the case of the
patients whose time course of recovery has been plotted.

Statistical Method of Analysis of the Data

The fact that descriptions of the neural and mental states of every patient were
not recorded in the hospital notes for each stated interval of time after injury
chosen for the study of the rate of recovery, presented a problem in the
transfer of data for computer-assisted statistical analysis. The rate of recovery

as an indicator of the long-term prognosis could not therefore be adequately examined by this method.

Information which was available in every case and which could be examined by statistical techniques included the most impaired state of neurological function recorded after admission to hospital (that is the maximum central neural disability score of the scale already defined), the duration of post-traumatic amnesia (also recorded in the hospital notes), the duration of coma, and, with certain qualifications as to type which have already been discussed in an earlier chapter, the duration of decerebration. Finally, although not available in every case, the rate of recovery was examined by noting whether or not a stated level in the decline of the central neural or mental disability score had been reached by a stated time in the case of every patient for whom the information had been recorded.

Suggestions for prediction were made by examining the relative numbers of patients whose central neural disabilities 10–25 years after injury had been scored as 1 or less (minimal or less), 1.5–2 (slight to moderate) and 2.5 or more (severe or worse) on the disability scale already defined. In table 13.1 the relationship between this triple classification of final outcome and maximum central neural disability score recorded after admission to hospital (that is, the worst state of neural responsiveness reached) and the duration of post-traumatic amnesia recorded in the hospital notes are set out. Where the triple classification clearly favours one outcome rather than the other two, the combination of the initial criteria of severity defining the subgroups of patients is evidently of value in predicting the long-term outcome.

It is at once apparent that prediction in the three age groups is different. Merely to be younger gives better prospects. Of the first two criteria of severity, the maximum central neural disability score seems more immediately useful in long-term prediction than the length of the post-traumatic amnesia. It cannot be improved upon in this consecutive series of patients for those injured between the ages of five and fifteen with a maximum central neural disability score of up to 4.5 or for those injured between the ages of sixteen and thirty-five with a maximum central neural disability score of up to 4. In the remaining groups of patients the distribution in the triple classification of outcome suggests that prediction by age and maximum central neural disability score might be improved upon. The length of post-traumatic amnesia is therefore considered as an additional indicator of long-term outcome, and the two groups in which it appears to be of value are shown in table 13.2. Here it may be seen that patients injured between the ages of sixteen and thirty-five with a maximum central neural disability score of 4.5 and 5, who had a post-traumatic amnesia of less than 9 weeks, are unlikely to be left with permanent central neural disability graded severe or worse, and in most cases the patient will be left with disability graded slight or less. In contrast a post-traumatic amnesia extending for 9 weeks or more in this same group of patients is highly likely to foreshadow long-term central neural

Table 13.1 Numbers of patients with final outcome central neural disability score as 0.5–1/1.5–2/2.5 or more (Minimal or less/Slight or Moderate/Severe or Worse) classified by age, maximum CND score after injury, and length of PTA

Age (years)	PTA (weeks)	Up to 4 (confused)	Maximum CND score 4.5 (semi-purposive or purposive)	5 (decerebrate)	Total
5–15	1–	5/ 0/ 0	6/ 0/ 0		11/ 0/ 0
	2–	4/ 0/ 0	10/ 0/ 0	1/ 1/ 0	15/ 1/ 0
	3–		4/ 0/ 1	2/ 0/ 0	6/ 0/ 1
	4–		1/ 0/ 0	1/ 1/ 0	2/ 1/ 0
	5–			6/ 1/ 1	6/ 1/ 1
	9–			1/ 1/ 0	1/ 1/ 0
	13+			0/ 1/ 0	0/ 1/ 0
	Total	9/ 0/ 0	21/ 0/ 1	11/ 5/ 1	41/ 5/ 2
16–35	1–	25/ 0/ 0	20/ 0/ 1	2/ 0/ 0	47/ 0/ 1
	2–	13/ 0/ 0	14/ 3/ 0	1/ 1/ 1	28/ 4/ 1
	3–	7/ 0/ 0	12/ 1/ 1	3/ 1/ 0	22/ 2/ 1
	4–	1/ 0/ 0	6/ 2/ 1	1/ 1/ 1	8/ 3/ 2
	5–	1/ 0/ 0	3/ 2/ 1	6/ 3/ 0	10/ 5/ 1
	9–	1/ 0/ 0	1/ 0/ 0	0/ 0/ 4	2/ 0/ 4
	13+		0/ 0/ 2	2/ 0/ 8	2/ 0/10
	Total	48/ 0/ 0	56/ 8/ 6	15/ 6/14	119/14/20
36 or over	1–	15/ 2/ 1	5/ 0/ 0		20/ 2/ 1
	2–	8/ 1/ 0	7/ 2/ 0	1/ 0/ 0	16/ 3/ 0
	3–	1/ 1/ 0	3/ 3/ 1		4/ 4/ 1
	4–	2/ 3/ 0	3/ 1/ 0	0/ 0/ 1	5/ 4/ 1
	5–	3/ 4/ 0	3/ 2/ 2	0/ 0/ 1	6/ 6/ 3
	9–		1/ 0/ 1	0/ 1/ 1	1/ 1/ 2
	13+		0/ 2/ 0	0/ 2/ 6	0/ 4/ 6
	Total	29/11/ 1	22/10/ 4	1/ 3/ 9	52/24/14
Total over all ages		86/11/ 1	99/18/11	27/14/24	212/43/36

Consecutive series, total 291.

disability graded severe or worse. Similarly, patients over the age of thirty-six at the time they were injured with a maximum central neural disability score after admission to hospital of 4.5 (that is, all but the decerebrate), and a post-traumatic amnesia of less than 3 weeks, are likely to have little long-term neural disability. In contrast, where the post-traumatic amnesia in the same group of patients has extended for longer than 3 weeks, long-term neural disability is more likely to be slight or worse.

An attempt was made to study the contribution to prediction of the long-term outcome provided by the rate of recovery. This was done by looking for improvement upon the accuracy of prediction already established

Table 13.2   Numbers of patients with final outcome central neural disability scores as in table 13.1, classified by selected lengths of PTA (showing only those groups from table 13.1 in which PTA appears to improve prediction)

Age	PTA (weeks)	Maximum CND score	
		4.5 and 5 (semi-purposive or purposive and decerebrate)	up to (including) 4.5 (all except decerebrate)
16–35	1–8	68/14/ 6	
	9+	3/ 0/14	
Totals		71/14/20	
36 or	1–2		35/ 5/ 1
over	3+		16/16/ 4
Totals			51/21/ 5

for the maximum central neural disability score (the worst state of neural responsiveness reached after admission to hospital), and the duration of post-traumatic amnesia. The time until the central neural disability score or the mental disability score either (a) fell to 3 (walking unassisted, and comprehending respectively), or (b) fell by a score of 1 or 1.5, was examined to establish whether there was any further improvement in prediction possible in four groups of patients. These were patients for whom the duration of post-traumatic amnesia had improved on the prediction given by central neural disability scores alone (shown in table 13.2), and patients injured between the ages of five and fifteen, or thirty-six and older, who had been decerebrate.

In patients injured between the ages of sixteen and thirty-five with a maximum central neural disability score of 4.5 or 5, and a post-traumatic amnesia of up to 2 months, there was a suggestion that those whose central neural disability score had not fallen by 1 by 1 month, or by 1.5 by 3 months, did worse and were likely to remain disabled by neural disability scored at 2.5 or more. In patients older than thirty-five at the time of injury with a maximum central neural disability score of 4 or less there was also a suggestion that those whose score had fallen more than 1.5 by 3 weeks had a substantially greater chance of being left with minimal or negligible central neural disability in the long-term.

Only in the case of patients injured between the ages of sixteen and thirty-five was it possible to show that predicting the outcome could be improved upon by using duration of decerebration in addition to maximum central neural disability score and duration of post-traumatic amnesia. This is shown in table 13.3.

The same procedure and triple classification are used in table 13.4 to examine the relationship between maximum mental disability score after injury, duration of post-traumatic amnesia and age, and the degree of mental disability found at review. In table 13.5 are shown these groups of patients in

Table 13.3 Numbers of patients with final outcome central neural disability scores as in table 13.1 aged between sixteen and thirty-five, with maximum CND score 4.5 or 5, classified by length of decerebration

PTA (weeks)	Decerebration	5 (decerebrate only)	4.5 (decerebrate and semi-purposive or purposive)
Up to 8	None or 1 day	9/ 1/ 1	64/ 9/ 5
	2 or more days	3/ 5/ 0	3/ 5/ 1
9 or more	None or 1 day	1/ 0/ 3	3/ 0/ 3
	2 or more days	0/ 0/11	0/ 0/11

Table 13.4 Numbers of patients with final outcome mental disability score as 1 or less/1.5 or 2/2.5 or more (Minimal or less/Slight or Moderate/Severe or Worse) classified by age, maximum MD score after injury and length of PTA

Age (years)	PTA (weeks)	Maximum MD score Up to 4 (confused)	4.5 (semi-purposive or purposive)	5 (decerebrate)	Total
5–15	1–	4/ 1/ 0	5/ 1/ 0		9/ 2/ 0
	2–	4/ 0/ 0	7/ 3/ 0	1/ 0/ 1	12/ 3/ 1
	3–		3/ 2/ 0	2/ 0/ 0	5/ 2/ 0
	4–		1/ 0/ 0	1/ 1/ 0	2/ 1/ 0
	5–			1/ 7/ 0	1/ 7/ 0
	9–			1/ 0/ 1	1/ 0/ 1
	13+			0/ 0/ 1	0/ 0/ 1
Total		8/ 1/ 0	16/ 6/ 0	6/ 8/ 3	30/15/ 3
16–35	1–	20/ 7/ 3	13/ 3/ 0	0/ 2/ 0	33/12/ 3
	2–	13/ 3/ 1	5/ 7/ 1	1/ 1/ 1	19/11/ 3
	3–	6/ 3/ 0	5/ 7/ 0	1/ 2/ 1	12/12/ 1
	4–	1/ 1/ 0	3/ 4/ 1	1/ 2/ 0	5/ 7/ 1
	5–	0/ 1/ 0	0/ 5/ 1	1/ 5/ 3	1/11/ 4
	9–	0/ 1/ 0	0/ 1/ 0	0/ 1/ 3	0/ 3/ 3
	13+		0/ 0/ 2	0/ 0/10	0/ 0/12
Total		40/16/ 4	26/27/ 5	4/13/18	70/56/27
36 or over	1–	12/ 6/ 0	3/ 2/ 0		15/ 8/ 0
	2–	3/ 6/ 2	1/ 5/ 1	1/ 0/ 0	5/11/ 3
	3–	1/ 1/ 0	0/ 7/ 0		1/ 8/ 0
	4–	2/ 2/ 1	2/ 1/ 1	0/ 0/ 1	4/ 3/ 3
	5–	0/ 3/ 4	1/ 2/ 4	1/ 0/ 0	2/ 5/ 8
	9–		0/ 1/ 2	0/ 0/ 1	0/ 1/ 3
	13+		0/ 0/ 2	0/ 0/ 8	0/ 0/10
Total		18/18/ 7	7/18/10	2/ 0/10	27/36/27
Total over all ages		66/35/11	49/51/15	12/21/31	127/107/57

Consecutive series, total 291.

Table 13.5   Numbers of patients with final outcome mental disability scores as in table 13.4, classified by selected lengths of PTA (showing only those groups in which PTA appears to improve prediction)

Age	PTA (weeks)	Maximum MD score	Number of patients
16–35	1– 2 or more	4.5	13/ 3/ 0 13/24/ 5
16–35	1– 9 or over	5	4/12/ 5 0/ 1/13
36 or over	1– 5 or over	4.5	6/15/ 2 1/ 3/ 8

whom prediction using duration of post-traumatic amnesia improves on the prediction based on maximum mental disability score.

It therefore seems that prediction of the long-term outcome of central neural and mental disability after severe accidental head injury may be made in retrospect with some accuracy and within a few weeks of the injury taking into account only three variables, namely age at the time of injury, the most impaired level of neurological responsiveness during the acute period after injury, and the duration of post-traumatic amnesia. The rate of recovery as an indicator of prognosis could not be examined adequately by this method because the data were incomplete, but there was some evidence to support the value of this measure suggested by the graphically illustrated recovery curves based on the information that was available.

Sequential Assessment

It is clear that a number of the variables used in this analysis to predict long-term outcome are interdependent. For this reason a sequential application of each in the assessment of its contribution to the accuracy of prediction appears a more appropriate method of analysis than, assuming independence of the variables as do Jennett and his colleagues, an examination of the frequency with which each is associated with different classes of outcome.

The prediction procedure implied by tables 13.1, 13.2 and 13.3 has therefore been drawn up in the form of 'flow diagrams', in figure 13.6 for the prediction of central neural disability, and figure 13.7 for the prediction of mental disability. Correct prediction of these three classes of outcome has been made in 90 per cent of cases for long-term central neural disability, and in 74 per cent for long-term mental disability in this consecutive series of patients. The confidence with which each outcome has been predicted by this procedure has been designated 'strong', 'moderate' or 'weak' on an arbitrary assessment of the extent of correct classification using these data. The

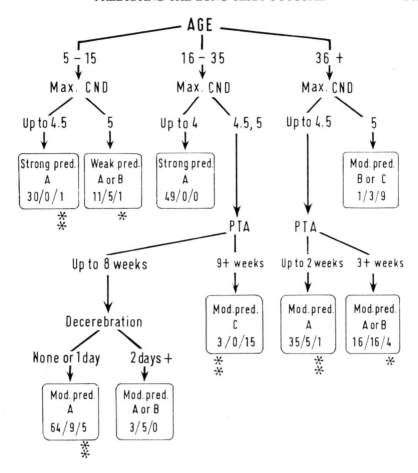

Figure 13.6   Predictive procedure for long-term outcome of central neural disability using only age at injury, worst state of neural responsiveness after injury (Max. CND), duration of PTA and duration of decerebration for the consecutive series of 291 patients (* and ** see tables 13.6, 13.7).

predictions A, B and C correspond to the same classes of final disability: A, 0.5 or 1 or less (minimal or less); B, 1.5 or 2 (slight or moderate); and C, 2.5 or more (severe or worse) as are used in the triple classification of the data. The paths through the procedure were established by inspection of the data. All branchings denote divisions into two groups with statistical significance of $P =$ 0.01 or stronger (usually much stronger). The procedure allows for interaction between the three predictors.

There was serious misclassification of long-term central neural disability in the case of 10 patients; that is, seven patients predicted minimally or not disabled in the long-term were severely disabled or worse, and three patients predicted severely disabled or worse were found to be minimally disabled. In addition there were five patients predicted moderately or slightly disabled or

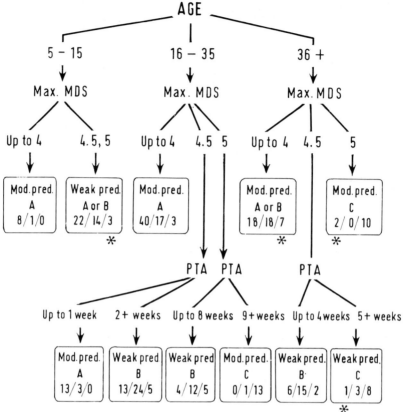

Figure 13.7   Predictive procedure for long-term outcome of mental disability using only age at injury, worst state of neural responsiveness after injury (Max. MDS), and duration of PTA for the consecutive series of 291 patients.

better who were found to be severely disabled or worse. The individual patients were identified and their disabilities are examined in detail in tables 13.6 and 13.7. The implications of these misclassifications and the way in which most would have been avoided by detailed clinical assessment of the individual in convalescence are discussed later. In the prediction of long-term mental disability there were nine serious misclassifications, that is by two grades, and seven others less seriously misclassified by only one grade as being less severely disabled than they turned out to be. The cases are examined in tables 13.6–13.9.

    The same prediction method has been applied to the selected series of Army and Addenbrooke's patients in figures 13.8 and 13.9. In this series of patients all were in coma longer than a month, and therefore by this criterion more severely injured than all but 24 of the consecutive series of patients on which the prediction procedure has been based. Correct prediction of the three classes of outcome of central neural disability was made in 72 per cent of

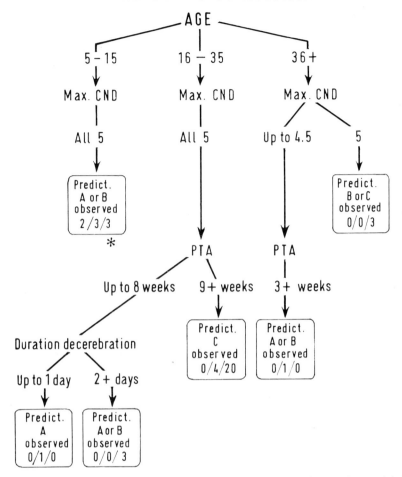

Figure 13.8 Predictive procedure for long-term outcome of central neural injury
using only age at injury, worst state of neural responsiveness after injury
(Max. CND), duration of PTA and duration of decerebration for the
selected series of 40 patients (Army and Addenbrooke's only).

cases, and of mental disability in 70 per cent of cases. The individual
characteristics of the disabilities in each of the six cases misclassified as to
central neural disability, and each of the four misclassified as to mental
disability are also examined in tables 13.6 and 13.7.

The Individual Patients Incorrectly Predicted

In tables 13.6–13.9 the specific disabilities of the ten patients seriously
misclassified as less or more disabled physically than they were found to be are
briefly described.

It may be seen from table 13.6 that four patients seriously misclassified by

Table 13.6 Individual patients whose long-term central neural disability was more severe than that incorrectly predicted using age at injury, worst state of neural response, durations of PTA and decerebration

Age	Initials and case number	CND score		
		Max.	Final	
Consecutive series				
5–15	**PJ 170	4.5	3	Dense hemiplegia. Walking unassisted 3 weeks.
	*RJ 054	5	3	Dense hemiplegia. Walking unassisted 3 months.
16–35	**WW 110C	4.5	3	Dense hemiplegia. Walking unassisted 2 months.
	**AM 066C	5	3	Dense hemiplegia. Walking unassisted 5 weeks.
	**PJ 156	4.5	2.5	Moderate hemiplegia. Walking unassisted 6 weeks.
	**WA 187	4.5	2.5	Moderate hemiplegia. Walking unassisted 6 weeks.
	**SB 213	4.5	2.5	Moderate hemiplegia. Walking unassisted 6 weeks.
36–45	**RT 042	4	3	Dense hemiplegia. Walking unassisted 3 months.
46–55	*JW 129	4.5	2.5	Slight brainstem cerebellar syndrome + severe disequilibrium. Walking unassisted 2 months.
	*CD 286	4.5	2.5	Slight brainstem cerebellar syndrome. Severe disequilibrium. Walking unassisted 6 weeks.
	*DL 063C	4.5	2.5	Moderately severe brainstem cerebellar syndrome. Walking unassisted 5 weeks.
	*RB 146C	4.5	3	Dense hemiplegia. Walking unassisted 3 months.
Selected series: Army and Cambridge				
5–15	*PB 056	5	3	Dense hemiplegia.
	*PH 058	5	3.5	Dense paraplegia.
	*EP 053	5	4.5	Decerebrate dementia.
16–25	*TK 027	5	2.5	Despite PTA only 8 weeks not walking till 6 weeks.
	*WC 001	5	3	Despite PTA only 8 weeks not walking unassisted till 3 months.
	*PR 054	5	2.5	Despite PTA only 8 weeks not walking unassisted till 2 months.

** Misclassified two grades of severity of disability.
 * Misclassified one grade less severely disabled than observed.

Table 13.7 Individual patients whose long-term mental disability was more severe than that incorrectly predicted using age at injury, worst state of neural response, durations of PTA and decerebration

Age	Initials and case number	MD score Max.	Final	
Consecutive series				
5–15	**YS 097	5	2.5	Severe frontolimoic dementia + slight brainstem cerebellar syndrome.
	**RS 109	5	2.5	Constitutional subnormality + slight brainstem cerebellar syndrome.
	**JA 050	5	3	Intractable epilepsy causing progressive personality deterioration.
16–35	**DH 144C	3	2.5	Indecent exposure recidivist. No neural disability.
	**MB 027	3	2.5	Recurrent anxiety depressions with defective memory. No neural disability.
	**LP 082C	4	3.5	Intractable epilepsy with progressive paranoid dementia.
36–45	*WL 147	3.5	2.5	Recurrent endogenous depressions. Negligible neural disability.
	*JC 207	3.5	2.5	Chronic anxiety depression. No neural disability.
	*DC 169	4	2.5	?Psychopath before and since. Negligible neural disability.
55+	*LH 279	3.5	3	Mild dementia and severely paranoid. ?Paraphrenia.
	*GF 212	3	4	Mild dementia and severely paranoid. ?Paraphrenia.
	*DB 115	4	3	Static slight dementia with phobic depressions since.
	*HH 258	3	2.5	Static slight dementia with phobic depressions since.
Selected series: Army and Cambridge				
5–15	*EP 053	5	4.5	Decerebrate dementia.
	*JB 044	5	2.5	Moderate frontolimbic dementia with still improving brainstem cerebellar syndrome at 5 years.
	*PB 056	5	3.5	Aphasic severe athetoid pseudobulbar syndrome.
	*PH 058	4.5	3	Frontolimbic dementia severe with dense paraplegia.

** Misclassified two grades of severity of disability.
 * Misclassified one grade less severely disabled than observed.

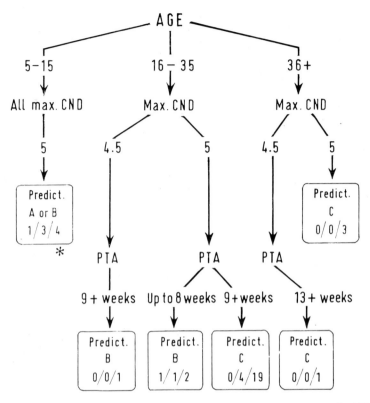

Figure 13.9   Predictive procedure for long-term outcome of mental disability using only age at injury, worst state of neural responsiveness after injury (Max. CND) and duration of PTA for the selected series of 40 patients (Army and Addenbrooke's only).

two grades of disability in the consecutive series had dense hemipareses so severe as to preclude normal domestic, social or occupational life. This was the cause of profound disability which had not been predicted either by the worst state of neurological responsiveness or the duration of post-traumatic amnesia. There were three other young adults still severely disabled by their pareses to degrees which seriously limited but did not preclude normal life in these three spheres, who were also seriously misclassified on the basis of these two indices. Only the child was walking unassisted within a month of the injury. Therefore on this predictive criterion, that is, the rate of recovery of central neural disability, only he would have been seriously misclassified. Individual assessment at 3 and 6 months and at a year had in every case shown the persisting pareses to be unchanged, as they remained more than 10 years later. All of these patients had cortical sensory deficits in the paralysed limbs as evidence, already discussed, that the pathology was likely to have been ischaemic and focal rather than diffuse and traumatic. This seems the probable explanation of the underestimation of long-term disability by the criteria of the worst level of neurological dysfunction and the duration of post-traumatic amnesia alone. The remaining three patients whose neural disabilities were found to be one grade worse than predicted were all older than forty-six at the time they were injured. The severe imbalance which continued to disable each of them had been evident in convalescence at 3 months.

Of the three children seriously misclassified in the selected series one was the only patient surviving nearly 10 years in a state of decerebrate dementia from either series, and both the other two patients were so severely disabled by pseudobulbar neural lesions that one was only beginning to walk unassisted at the end of a year, and the other remained permanently chairbound by his spastic paraparesis. In other words all three children would have been correctly predicted if assessed individually in convalescence on the basis of their slow rate of recovery and the pattern of their lesions. Similarly, in the case of the three adults, unassisted walking was delayed to an extent which correlated well with their final disability scores.

There were only three cases incorrectly predicted two grades of disability as being more disabled by their central neural lesions than they turned out to be. These are shown in table 13.8. Misclassification in each was due to the fact

Table 13.8 Individual patients from the consecutive series whose long-term central neural disability was less severe (by two grades) than that incorrectly predicted using age at injury, worst state of neural response, durations of PTA and decerebration

Age	Initials and case number	CND score		
		Max.	Final	
16–35	PT 179	4.5	1	PTA 9 weeks with dysphasia which improved.
	AP 285	4	0.5	PTA 9 weeks. Frontal personality change and memory impairment.
	PM 121C	5	1	PTA 9 weeks. Frontal personality change.

that the post-traumatic amnesia extended for longer than 2 months, foreshadowing persisting intellectual impairment or personality change in all, but only slight central neural disability. This was despite the fact that unassisted walking was delayed for over a month in each of them. In other words in these three individuals neurophysical recovery was ultimately better than could have been predicted even after assessment of the individual case in convalescence. In retrospect it is not apparent why this should have been so.

In table 13.7 the individual patients misclassified as to mental disability are examined. Intractable epilepsy with progressive personality deterioration accounts for two misclassifications. In neither case was this eventuality predictable within a year of the injury, either on the basis of the four indices of long-term outcome already examined or the character of the epilepsy. One of the children was undoubtedly a constitutional dullard, and this may explain in part the persisting high mental disability score. The other child remained with a greater degree of frontolimbic personality change than was usually seen in the children. In her case coma had lasted a month, decerebration 3 days, and she had not been able to walk unassisted until 2 months after the injury. Her residual neural disabilities were slight, as was the case generally with most of the children, but she remained childish, disinhibited and was having difficulty in holding down her job as a ward maid 16 years after her injury. The predictive criteria did not suggest the personality aberration which resulted in repeated imprisonment for indecent exposure of one of the adolescents, nor the recurrent disabling anxiety depressions of the other. None of the selected series was seriously misclassified by two grades with respect to long-term mental disability. In table 13.9 are shown the three older patients predicted as

Table 13.9 Individual patients from the consecutive series whose long-term mental disability was less severe (by two grades) than that incorrectly predicted using age at injury, worst state of neural response, durations of PTA and decerebration

Age	Initials and case number	MD score		
		Max.	Final	
36–45	ET 088C	5	1	
	AB 095	5	2	Severe brainstem cerebellar syndrome.
	AM 215	4.5	2	Probable incorrect assumption of constitutional mental subnormality because husband was mentally defective.

being more disabled by two grades than they were. It can only be said of these that one was quite unaccountably less disabled, another had predictably severe central neural disability, but not the expected associated mental disability, and the third was almost certainly incorrectly assumed to be constitutionally mentally subnormal, as was her husband who, in consequence, provided a none too helpful independent account.

Referring again to table 13.6, there was incorrect prediction of central neural disability, in which the outcome was only one grade worse than predicted, in the case of five individuals from the consecutive series. The child and one of the adults were left with severe hemipareses, the child failing to walk unassisted until 6 months, and the adult until 3 months. One of the other adults was walking at 5 weeks unassisted, but in the case of the other two, walking without assistance was delayed for 6 weeks and 2 months.

Prediction of mental disability (in patients from the consecutive series) which proved to be incorrect by one grade (table 13.7) was found to be due to chronic anxiety depressions in the case of two patients, and what might well have been constitutional psychopathy in another. The remaining four patients from the consecutive series were aged fifty-five years or older at the time of injury and two of these were disabled by a progressively worsening paranoid dementia, and two by a mild static dementia associated with symptoms of anxiety and depression.

The four patients from the selected, and more seriously injured, series, whose mental disability was incorrectly predicted by one grade, included the three children already described with neurophysical disabilities so profoundly disabling that they would have been correctly identified had they been assessed individually in convalescence. In the case of the other child, whose defective intellectual functions were still more disabling than predicted when she was re-examined 5 years after her injury, it was clear that the neurophysical disabilities had improved sufficiently in the preceding 2 years to allow reclassification in a lower disability grade. It is probable that, as with the rest of the series, the improvement in mental disability was lagging behind the improvement in central neural disability, and that within the 10 years, which is the shortest period for which the majority were followed up, there could be further improvement in her intellectual abilities and finally a lower mental disability score.

Summary of Prediction Guide

Children whose injury has not caused decerebration will do very well in the long-term and be left with little or no neurophysical disability. If they have been decerebrate, most will still have little, or only slight to moderate, central neural or mental disability ultimately unless the injury has caused brain damage of a degree usually incompatible with life. These cases will be only too easily identified within 3 months of the injury. It follows that despite apparently profound degrees of impaired neural function in the acute stage after injury the long-term outlook is good for children given time, and a poor prognosis for neural or mental disability should not be assumed within 3 or even perhaps 5 years of the injury. Even then the problems of adolescence may well suggest a continuing personality disorder which will not persist, at least to a profoundly disabling extent, into adult life.

Adolescents and young adults will all recover without neural disability if no more than confused after their injury. There is a greater chance of slight to moderate memory impairment or personality change persisting, but this will rarely be severely disabling. Those whose level of neurological function after injury has been reduced to purposive or decerebrate response to stimulation and who have up to 2 months' PTA, and one day's decerebration, will seldom be disabled. Those with longer PTA and/or decerebration will be moderately or, more commonly, severely or profoundly disabled by their neural lesions. A PTA of 2–8 weeks after similar degrees of disturbed neural function in the acute stage after injury will usually result in moderate disability by memory impairment or personality change. Those decerebrate with a PTA of more than 2 months will be severely disabled or worse both mentally and by their central neural lesions.

The middle-aged and older who were not decerebrate, and whose PTA was no more than a fortnight, will nearly all have no neurophysical disability, but of those who were decerebrate most will have severe disability. Decerebration over the age of 46 at the time of injury is not usually survived for any length of time. Mental disability is commoner at this age after an injury causing a PTA of 1 week or more, but severely disabling degrees are unlikely in those no more than confused initially. Where the level of impairment of neural function after injury is reduced to purposive or semi-purposive response to stimulation, a PTA of less than 1 month is seldom associated with more than moderate mental or central neural disability. More than 1 month's PTA in these patients is likely to be followed by severe degrees of mental disability. Decerebration following injury sustained after the age of 35 is almost invariably followed by severe mental disability.

Predicting the Time until Return to Work

The relationship between the time away from work, or failure to return to any form of gainful employment, and the three predictive criteria of age, worst state of neurological responsiveness, and duration of post-traumatic amnesia is set out in table 13.10. It may be seen that prediction on the basis of these three indices again provides an accurate general guide. The question of the extent to which central neural and mental disabilities have resulted in a decline in work status has already been examined in an earlier chapter. The effect of head injury on gainful employment was an integral part of the assessment of overall disability taken into account in the scoring method used to grade long-term disabilities. It is self-evident that how often the more seriously disabled can be found gainful employment will be affected by levels of employment in the general population, and that therefore this exercise in prediction of long-term outcome depends to a considerable extent upon factors which cannot be taken into account in study of this kind. It can none the less be seen that in general these three predictive indices do provide a guide to the likelihood or otherwise of gainful employment in the long-term after the severest forms of accidental head injury in civil life. For example in the combined series of 331 patients 33 of 36 adults who had been decerebrate with a post-traumatic amnesia of 13 weeks or more were never gainfully employed again, though 3 of the 5 children were. In contrast, of those adults no more than confused after injury and with a post-traumatic amnesia of less than 2 weeks, 36 of 43 were back at work within 3 months, and all the children were back at school by this time.

The likelihood that anyone will succeed in improving his occupational status after a head injury of this severity seems to be relatively slight. It may be seen from table 13.11 that only 16 out of 291, that is about 6 per cent, of the consecutive series of patients, were assessed as having made a change in their occupational status after their injuries which could be considered an improve-

Table 13.10   Numbers of patients with time to return to work/school, classified as up to 3 months/4–6 months/7 months +/unemployed or sheltered work, by age, maximum CND score after injury, and PTA

Age (years)	PTA (weeks)	Maximum CND score			Total
		Up to 4 (confused)	4.5 (semi-purposive or purposive)	5 (decerebrate)	
5–15	1–	4/ 1/ 0/ 0	3/ 1/ 1/ 0		7/ 2/ 1/ 0
	2–	3/ 1/ 0/ 0	4/ 5/ 1/ 1	0/ 0/ 1/ 1	7/ 6/ 2/ 2
	3–		3/ 1/ 0/ 1	1/ 1/ 0/ 0	4/ 2/ 0/ 1
	4–		1/ 0/ 0/ 0	0/ 2/ 0/ 0	1/ 2/ 0/ 0
	5–			0/ 5/ 6/ 0	0/ 5/ 6/ 0
	9–			0/ 1/ 1/ 1	0/ 1/ 1/ 1
	13+			0/ 0/ 2/ 3	0/ 0/ 2/ 3
Total		7/ 2/ 0/ 0	11/ 7/ 2/ 2	1/ 9/10/ 5	19/18/12/ 7
16–35	1–	10/12/ 3/ 0	10/ 6/ 5/ 0	0/ 2/ 0/ 0	20/20/ 8/ 0
	2–	5/ 2/ 4/ 2	5/ 7/ 5/ 0	2/ 0/ 0/ 1	12/ 9/ 9/ 3
	3–	3/ 2/ 2/ 0	1/ 5/ 8/ 0	0/ 0/ 4/ 0	4/ 7/14/ 0
	4–	0/ 1/ 0/ 0	2/ 1/ 5/ 1	0/ 2/ 0/ 1	2/ 4/ 5/ 2
	5–	0/ 0/ 1/ 0	0/ 1/ 4/ 1	0/ 2/ 9/ 2	0/ 3/14/ 3
	9–	0/ 0/ 1/ 0	0/ 0/ 2/ 0	0/ 0/ 5/ 7	0/ 0/ 8/ 7
	13+		0/ 0/ 0/ 2	0/ 0/ 2/23	0/ 0/ 2/25
Total		18/17/11/ 2	18/20/29/ 4	2/ 6/20/34	38/43/60/40
36 or over	1–	11/ 3/ 2/ 2	3/ 0/ 0/ 2		14/ 3/ 2/ 4
	2–	2/ 6/ 1/ 0	2/ 3/ 2/ 2	1/ 0/ 0/ 0	5/ 9/ 3/ 2
	3–	0/ 1/ 1/ 0	0/ 2/ 2/ 3		0/ 3/ 3/ 3
	4–	0/ 1/ 2/ 2	0/ 3/ 1/ 0	0/ 0/ 0/ 1	0/ 4/ 3/ 3
	5–	0/ 2/ 0/ 5	1/ 2/ 4/ 0	0/ 0/ 1/ 0	1/ 4/ 5/ 5
	9–		0/ 0/ 1/ 1	0/ 0/ 1/ 1	0/ 0/ 2/ 2
	13+		0/ 0/ 0/ 3	0/ 0/ 1/10	0/ 0/ 1/13
Total		13/13/ 6/ 9	6/10/10/11	1/ 0/ 3/12	20/23/19/32
Total over all ages		38/32/17/11	35/37/41/17	4/15/33/51	77/84/91/79

Consecutive and selected series, total 331.

ment. This was seen in only one case where the post-traumatic amnesia had exceeded 3 weeks.

Discussion

The problem of predicting the ultimate disability to be expected after accidental head injury has provided a fruitful field for informed guesswork based on the anecdotal evidence of clinical experience and inappropriate comparisons with brain-damaged war wounded. In the last decade there has been an increasing number of studies attempting to gather more factual information about the long-term effects of severe brain injury sustained in

Table 13.11   Numbers of patients with occupational status as decline/unchanged/rise, classified by age, maximum CND score after injury, and length of PTA

Age (years)	PTA (weeks)	Maximum CND score			Total
		Up to 4 (confused)	4.5 (semi-purposive or purposive)	5 (decerebrate)	
5–15	1–	1/ 4/ 0	2/ 4/ 0		3/ 8/ 0
	2–	0/ 4/ 0	3/ 7/ 0	1/ 1/ 0	4/12/ 0
	3–		2/ 3/ 0	1/ 1/ 0	3/ 4/ 0
	4–		1/ 0/ 0	1/ 1/ 0	2/ 1/ 0
	5–			5/ 3/ 0	5/ 3/ 0
	9–			1/ 1/ 0	1/ 1/ 0
	13+			1/ 0/ 0	1/ 0/ 0
Total		1/ 8/ 0	8/14/ 0	10/ 7/ 0	19/29/ 0
16–35	1–	3/19/ 3	2/16/ 3	1/ 1/ 0	6/36/ 6
	2–	3/ 9/ 1	5/ 8/ 4	1/ 2/ 0	9/19/ 5
	3–	1/ 6/ 0	5/ 8/ 1	3/ 1/ 0	9/15/ 1
	4–	0/ 1/ 0	5/ 4/ 0	1/ 2/ 0	6/ 7/ 0
	5–	0/ 1/ 0	4/ 1/ 1	6/ 3/ 0	10/ 5/ 1
	9–	1/ 0/ 0	1/ 0/ 0	3/ 1/ 0	5/ 1/ 0
	13+		2/ 0/ 0	10/ 0/ 0	12/ 0/ 0
Total		8/36/ 4	24/37/ 9	25/10/ 0	57/83/13
36 or over	1–	6/ 9/ 3	2/ 3/ 0		8/12/ 3
	2–	5/ 4/ 0	4/ 5/ 0	0/ 1/ 0	9/10/ 0
	3–	0/ 2/ 0	3/ 4/ 0		3/ 6/ 0
	4–	4/ 1/ 0	1/ 3/ 0	1/ 0/ 0	6/ 4/ 0
	5–	5/ 2/ 0	5/ 2/ 0	0/ 1/ 0	10/ 5/ 0
	9–		2/ 0/ 0	1/ 1/ 0	3/ 1/ 0
	13+		2/ 0/ 0	8/ 0/ 0	10/ 0/ 0
Total		20/18/ 3	19/17/ 0	10/ 3/ 0	49/38/ 3
Total over all ages		29/62/ 7	51/68/ 9	45/20/ 0	125/150/16

Consecutive series, total 291.

civil life. Selection criteria and methods of assessment in these studies most closely comparable with the present one were reviewed in an earlier chapter. There was a general consensus amongst them that outcome was closely related, first to the degree of disturbed neurological function seen in the acute stage after injury, second to the rate at which recovery of neurophysical disability took place, and third to the age at the time of injury. This is clear not only from the details of the individual reports but from the way in which it was possible to classify into three groups all the studies reviewed. The first had selected patients, most of them adults, judged severely injured mainly on the basis of indirect measures of severity which included the worst state of neurological dysfunction, or the durations of coma, confusion, decerebration and post-traumatic amnesia; the second dealt with patients who were still sufficiently disabled by their central neural lesions to require physiotherapeutic rehabilitation in convalescence; and the third were studies concerned solely with the somewhat different prognosis that appeared to be the sequel of head injuries of comparable severity in children.

The method of prediction outlined in the present chapter may have done little more than confirm the generalisations of these earlier studies. The data presented do, however, examine in detail the extent to which each measure of severity and age can be relied upon to give an accurate prediction of the long-term outcome, and they draw attention to the fact that, taken separately or sequentially, prediction based on these criteria alone should only be used as a general guide.

There cannot be any simple one-to-one relationship between the duration of coma or post-traumatic amnesia, or the state of disturbed neurological function in the acute stage after injury, and, say, marital harmony, or the extent to which social intercourse or employment will be affected in the individual case. Generalisations based on these criteria of severity of injury may well ignore the nature and degree of specific disabilities, and will fail to take account of the individual's response to the particular pattern of defective intellect or memory, personality change and physical disabilities he has suffered. The prerequisite for accurate long-term prediction in the individual case is a detailed knowledge of the residual patterns of mental and neurophysical disability which do persist long after severe brain injury. The recognition of these in convalescence, their degree, and the individual's response to them, can then be examined against the general guide given by the predictive criteria outlined above. It cannot be other than by the careful clinical assessment of the pattern of intellectual impairment, personality change and neurophysical disability in each patient that accurate prediction will be made. When these general predictions seem out of keeping with the progress of the individual patient an examination of possible sources of error is needed. Amongst these will be the individual's constitutional intelligence and personality, the severity of focal ischaemic neural lesions superimposed upon lesser degrees of overall mechanical brain trauma, the separate problems of optic and other cranial nerve lesions, the severity of the traumatic epilepsy, psychiatric illness precipitated but not in general to be expected in the majority after head injury, and finally simulation for gain.

The definition of classes of outcome presents considerable difficulty. The more specific the requirements for inclusion in each class, the more they are likely to ignore the remarkable extent to which acceptable or at least tolerable degrees of domestic, social or occupational rehabilitation can be achieved. In their classification of outcome, Jennett, Teasdale, Galbraith, Pickard, Grant, Braakman, Avezaat, Maas, Minderhoud, Vecht, Heiden, Small, Caton and Kurze (1977) report a high degree of accuracy of prediction of the short-term outcome based on a complex method of computer-assisted analysis of numerically-scored sequential clinical assessments made in the first few days after injury. They are able in this way to distinguish patients with the worst prognosis who will die or survive in 'persistent vegetative states', a third group who remain so severely disabled as to be incapable of managing without assistance at some time during a 24-hour period, a fourth group who are moderately disabled but capable of organising their own lives, travelling by public transport and working either in a sheltered environment or at a lower level, and the remainder who make a 'good recovery'.

In the present study it was apparent that the fact that there was some dependence on the spouse, a normal enough human state, and that without this an individual might not be able to get through 24 hours unaided, did not necessarily preclude a relatively normal domestic, social and occupational life in many instances. Similarly, an individual who could not use public transport was not invariably incapable of getting through 24 hours of the day and night unaided. Neither did the failure to resume all previous occupational and leisure pursuits mean that there had been severe damage to mental or central neural functions. Persisting positional vertigo, homonymous hemianopias and the occasional major fit often prevented the resumption of the previous occupation and the enjoyment of sporting activities but did not preclude a relatively normal although perhaps different job. Including individuals with these minor sequelae amongst those who can be employed only in a sheltered workshop illustrates some of the difficulties associated with assigning patients to specifically defined yet broad categories of outcome.

It is remarkable how little effect homonymous hemianopias and minor epilepsy will have on the lives of some people, for example the long-distance ammunition lorry driver who was so disabled, already referred to in an earlier chapter.

It may be argued that a classification of outcome which includes amongst the severely disabled who are not precluded from living relatively normal domestic, social or occupational lives all those who cannot get through 24 hours without some aid, is likely to be of less value than one which attempts to single out the special feature of some degree of dependence.

In fact the original classification attempted in the present study was designed to study more than simply the long-term outcome. Amongst other aspects of closed head injury the intention was to examine the relationship between minimal signs of pyramidal lesions and the side of head impact. Several of the 10 classes of outcome defined contained numbers of patients too small for useful computer-assisted analysis of the factors predicting outcome, and some elision was necessary. Within the severely disabled group of patients it would have been a relatively simple matter to identify in convalescence most of those whose degree of dependence had remained total. Of those not walking unaided by 3 months, only 14 out of 55, that is 25 per cent, were not totally disabled 10 or more years later, four of those being children and 10 adolescents. There were only two children and four adolescents amongst the 36 who were not walking unaided at 6 months, that is 11 per cent who did not remain totally and permanently dependent.

Rather than make one or more specific features of the final disability exclusive or inclusive in a particular class of outcome, it was felt important in the present study to use a more general measurement of disability. This would take account of the fact that, despite adequate domestic or social or occupational rehabilitation, or all three, the classification of outcome recognised the degree to which there was more or less disability in all or one of these spheres of activity. Similarly, at the other end of the scale, where superficially there was no alteration in domestic, social or occupational life, a mild forgetfulness, or increase in the level of anxiety or off-handedness, or minimal defects of articulation, balance and coordination or spasticity, although hardly disabling, could be allowed for. The triple classification of outcome in this study is as a result finer for lesser degrees of disability, and more inclusive for the more severe degrees than that employed in many of the papers already cited. Using the simple predictive indices generally available in retrospect in the records of even non-specialist hospitals, and an assessment of PTA which can be determined in retrospect, prediction into these classes of outcome was in general accurate. Within these broad categories of outcome it becomes possible, as convalescence progresses, to recognise specific mental, central neural, cranial nerve, and other disabilities which will persist in the long-term. But only by the sequential assessment of the individual patient after injury is it going to be justifiable to attempt to predict to what extent each disability is likely to persist, and to assess the most opportune time to introduce available techniques of physical or mental, occupational and social rehabilitation in each case.

14 Summary, Conclusions and Implications

In reviewing previous reports of the long-term outcome of severe head injury in civil life it became clear that age at the time of injury, the severity of the injury judged by indirect measures of the level of neurological responsiveness and the durations of decerebration, altered consciousness and post-traumatic amnesia, and also the rate of recovery from neurophysical disability seen by the need for admission to physiotherapeutic rehabilitation units, were all more or less closely related to prognosis. These were a heterogenous series of studies in which there was no consistent definition either of the concept of severe or of what constituted the long-term.

In order to provide a random, or more accurately a representative sample of severe cases of head injury for this epidemiological study, every patient amnesic or unconscious for 1 week or longer was identified in a population of 7000 admitted consecutively between 10 and 24 years earlier to one regional accident service. This service provided neurosurgical care of head injuries. All but 10 of these 479 cases were traced, the cause of death was established for 178 and the remaining 291 were followed up and examined. To enlarge the most severely injured group, a further selected series of 69 patients surviving injuries which had caused coma lasting a month or more between 3 and 25 years earlier was also studied. The cause of death was established in 28 of these, one was untraceable, and the remaining 40 were re-examined.

It became apparent that there were four readily recognisable patterns of neurological lesions that might persist indefinitely, and eight rather less clearly defined types of mental disability. Descriptions of similar syndromes were found in a number of the studies of long-term outcome after severe accidental head injury already referred to, and also in several reports concerned with other aspects of the subject. It seemed likely that on the basis of certain features of the clinical course, the site of head impact and its relationship to the lateralisation of signs of minor residual pyramidal lesions in the less severely injured, there were differences in the underlying pathological processes. This suggested that irreversible and untreatable mechanical effects of the injury were often less the cause of persistent disability than were potentially treatable secondary perfusion failure and brain swelling.

The fact that others concerned with the field of accidental head injury had observed similar post-traumatic syndromes also suggested the possibility of a readily communicated shorthand description of the types of residual disabilities which have to be dealt with in rehabilitation and compensation. It was clear that life expectancy was closely related to the pattern of the residual neural lesions. The majority of those who survived in states of 'decerebrate dementia' died within a year, and although small numbers might live a few years longer, only exceptionally would there be survival for a decade. In contrast, most of those with even the most severe forms of the 'athetoid pseudobulbar' syndrome, who recovered sufficiently to be discharged from hospital and walk without assistance, appeared to have little reduction of life expectancy except by epilepsy, accidental drowning or inhalation of food, and suicide. The remainder, with varying degrees of the 'brainstem cerebellar' or minor 'hemiparetic' pattern of lesions, who had recovered from the immediate effects of their injury and left hospital had no more than an overall 5-year reduction in life expectancy.

The degree of disability associated with each of these syndromes of central neural lesions was relatively constant. The cases of decerebrate dementia almost invariably required the resources of a ward in a hospital, although occasionally parents of young children managed with some professional or even non-professional assistance to provide adequate care at home for a period. Those with the athetoid pseudobulbar syndrome were commonly totally dependent upon others for most of their day-to-day needs, and required continuing care either from relatives or in more or less suitable homes and units for the chronically disabled. The associated intellectual impairment and personality change in these patients was usually also severely disabling and contributed to their total dependence. This was not the case in most patients with the brainstem cerebellar pattern of lesions, and even severe ataxia and impressive degrees of euphoria and disinhibition did not preclude a relatively acceptable domestic and social life though it might limit substantially most forms of gainful employment. The majority left with minimal signs of pyramidal lesions, of which they were not aware, were in no way disabled physically, though a number were by their personality change or defective memory. It was in these patients with the least evidence of permanent brain damage that there appeared to be greater impairment of intellectual functions, as assessed by psychometric tests, in those who had been struck on the right side of the head. This suggests a possible explanation for some as yet unexplored aspects of the post-concussional syndrome.

As the study progressed, patterns of persisting mental disability also emerged which, like the patterns of disabilities due to central neural lesions, were closely related to the severity of the injury and the age at which it had occurred. There were eight relatively clearly defined chronically disabling types of personality change with or without associated impairment of memory and intellectual functions which were seen repeatedly. Again all seemed to have been described, though in somewhat different terms reflecting the individual interests of the authors, in the extensive literature concerned with the mental after-effects of head injury. Descriptive titles intended to draw attention both to characteristic features of the type of mental disorder and the sites of brain injury these reflected were coined in order to provide a shorthand method of identification for comparison with other studies, and to save repetition. The most frequently encountered disabling pattern of 'frontolimbic dementia' was seen only after the severest forms of brain injury, and was virtually confined to adolescents and young adults. It was usually found with the athetoid pseudobulbar and severe brainstem cerebellar patterns of neural lesions. It consisted of various manifestations of frontal personality change together with profound impairment of day-to-day memory and the release of irritability and rage reactions. The latter, rather than dementia, were often the cause of the severest domestic, social and occupational disability. 'Frontal dysmnesia', and frontal personality change without memory impairment, and both without the release of irritability were rather commoner sequels of less severe injury in the young. Frontal personality change with pathological irritability, and also memory impairment and irritability without the personality changes of orbitofrontal injury were uncommon, and focal cognitive deficits, even dysphasia, were rare in the absence of dementia.

Two highly characteristic sequelae of injury after middle age were patterns of disability dominated by anxiety: 'dysmnesic inadequacy' apparently reflecting a neurotic response to memory and other less obvious cognitive deficits, and 'phobic imbalance' a neurotic reaction to various forms of traumatic vestibular disorder. In neither of these latter conditions was it usual to find other than minimal signs of central neural lesions. These two long-term sequelae of major head injury were seen therefore to bear a striking resemblance to the so-called post-concussional syndrome following minor concussive injury. 'Traumatic dysmnesia' alone, that is without personality change or other than minimal evidence of neural lesions, was another common long-term sequel of the relatively less severe injuries at all ages.

On the basis of the prevalence of seven cases of schizophreniform psychoses encountered in this study, the invariable association with dementia and the inconstant relationship to the severity of the head injury which preceded it, there were grounds for suggesting that 'traumatic paranoid dementia' more appropriately described the condition. Evidence that a schizophreniform illness in the absence of dementia was likely to be precipitated by severe head injury was slight. In contrast, depressive illnesses with the characteristics of endogenous affective disorders had clearly been precipitated by the head injury in 4 per cent of the consecutive series of patients. In a small number of these there was a substantial delay, almost certainly accounted for by the time taken for the early traumatic frontal personality change to regress. Suicide was three times as common as it is found in the general population. Decline in occupational status was more commonly due to mental than to neurophysical disability in all social classes with the exception of the unskilled manual worker.

In an examination of the prevalence of persisting impairment of cranial nerve functions it was found that the risks of permanent anosmia increased with age, rising to almost 50 per cent where injury had occurred over the age of forty-five. The relative infrequency with which evidence of other cranial nerve lesions was seen to persist is in keeping with previously reported studies of prevalence after closed head injury. In the case of optic nerve and chiasmal lesions the overall figure was 3 per cent for persisting visual field defects. Diplopia due to residual third nerve palsies was found in 7 per cent, and due to lateral rectus weakness in about 4 per cent of cases in the consecutive series of patients, the prevalence in both cases being slightly higher in complicated injuries. Neither the visual field defects nor the diplopia appeared to have constituted serious disability, and less than half a dozen patients had needed surgical correction for the diplopia. A sensory deficit due to trigeminal nerve injury was a rarity and there was not one case of post-traumatic neuralgia or causalgia. Complete facial nerve palsies were similarly rare. The prevalence of these and incomplete palsies with aberrant reinnervation was only 3 per cent. All those with persisting facial palsies had sustained fractured skulls. Mild degrees of impairment of hearing in one or both ears dating from injury were common complaints but total permanent loss of hearing in an ear was rare. Vertigo almost invariably took the form of transient sensations of rotation and imbalance provoked by movement. Nearly a quarter of the patients were still experiencing positional vertigo more than 10 years after injury, but neither age at the time of injury nor the type or severity of the head injury seemed related to its persistence.

In the case of headache no association with age, the type of head injury or its severity was found. Persistence of headache was closely related to its character and severity. It appeared that the more severe the headache and the more closely it assumed the characteristics of so-called vascular and migrainous headaches the more likely was it to last for longer than a year, and conversely, that the less severe the headache the more likely was it to clear up within months of the injury.

Despite the well-established fact that traumatic haemorrhage and infarction in the supra-optic region of the hypothalamus and adjacent infundibular region are an almost invariable finding in patients who die within days of their head injuries, the frequency with which impairment of pituitary or hypothalamic function was found in the survivors of the present series of patients was minimal. In contrast, the high incidence of transient hypothalamic hyperphagia and diabetes insipidus noted in the hospital records during convalescence confirms the frequency with which severe closed acceleration head injury is associated with hypothalamic damage seen in survivors. The relevance of this observation to the syndrome of released irritability and rage reactions so commonly seen after severe head injury seems obvious.

A progressive neuronal degeneration attributable to the cumulative effects of repeated minor head injury may occur in boxers which is not associated with the histological changes characteristic of normal ageing. In the present study there were no specific features in the head injuries of those who progressively demented either immediately or after a delay, which distinguished them from the rest of the sample, yet progressive intellectual deterioration was not a rare occurrence. If there were a specific neuronal degeneration provoked by a single head injury it seems unlikely that the pathology of such a relatively common condition would have been overlooked until now. The phenomenon of premature ageing of a brain already damaged by injury has been confirmed by others comparing the ageing of elderly injured patients with those in a psychiatric community who had not sustained head injuries. The normal effects of ageing upon a brain already depleted of its functional reserve by injury seems the most likely explanation for most cases of progressive intellectual deterioration observed in the present study, although the possibility of ageing processes being accelerated or perhaps even precipitated by injury remains to be investigated.

There was an overall prevalence of post-traumatic epilepsy of 28 per cent in the consecutive series. This varied from 7 per cent amongst those with an uncomplicated injury and a post-traumatic amnesia of no more than a week to 61 per cent in those whose injuries had been complicated by brain compression and traumatic or surgical penetration of brain substance. There was increasing prevalence of epilepsy with length of post-traumatic amnesia in uncomplicated injury, as there was in both complicated and uncomplicated injuries with duration of coma.

In the survivors re-examined from the consecutive series the epileptic attacks had become progressively less frequent in all but three patients. In the majority the attacks had also become abortive or minor variants of the earlier ones. There were no features of the epilepsy in the early stages which would have identified the three patients whose post-traumatic epilepsy was not benign, as it was in the majority, except that in each case once the attacks had begun they persisted as generalised convulsions which progressively increased in frequency despite treatment. There were four premature deaths directly related to traumatic epilepsy in the unselected series of patients, and two more patients sustained second severe head injuries during fits. The long-term natural history of post-traumatic epilepsy in accidental head injury appears therefore to be very similar to that which follows missile wounds of the brain. This is in marked contrast to the differences between the neurophysical and mental disabilities which follow these two distinct types of injury.

It was found that using only the age at injury and two indirect indices of severity of injury, the worst state of neurological responsiveness and the duration of post-traumatic amnesia, a generally accurate guide to long-term outcome was obtained.

Children whose injury has not caused decerebration will in the long term do very well and be left with little or no neurophysical disability. If they have been decerebrate, most will still have little or only slight to moderate central neural or mental disability ultimately, unless the injury has caused brain damage of a degree usually incompatible with life. These cases will be only too easily identified within 3 months of the injury. It follows that despite apparently profound degrees of impaired neural function in the acute stage after injury, the long-term outlook is good for children given time, and a poor prognosis for neural or mental disability should not be assumed within 3, or even perhaps 5 years of the injury. Even then the problems of adolescence may well suggest a continuing personality disorder which will not persist, at least to a severely disabling extent, into adult life.

Adolescents and young adults will all recover without neural disability if no more than confused after their injury. There is a greater chance of slight to moderate memory impairment or personality change persisting, but this will rarely be severely disabling. Those whose level of neurological function after injury has been reduced to purposive or decerebrate response to stimulation and who have no more than 2 months' PTA, and 1 day's decerebration, will seldom be physically disabled. Those with longer PTA and/or decerebration will be moderately or, more commonly, severely or profoundly disabled by their neural lesions. A PTA of 2–8 weeks after similar degrees of disturbed neural function in the acute stage following injury will usually result in moderate disability due to memory impairment or personality change. Those decerebrate with a PTA of more than 2 months will be severely disabled or worse both mentally and physically because of their central neural lesions.

The middle-aged and older who were not decerebrate, and whose PTA was no more than a fortnight, will nearly all have no neurophysical disability, but of those who were decerebrate most will have severe disability. Decerebration over the age of forty-six at injury is not usually survived for any length of time. Mental disability is commoner at this age after an injury causing a PTA of 1 week or more, but severely disabling degrees are unlikely in those no more than confused initially. Where the level of impairment of neural function after injury is reduced to purposive or semi-purposive response to stimulation, a PTA of up to 1 month is seldom associated with more than moderate mental or central neural disability. More than 1 month's PTA in these patients is likely to be followed by severe degrees of mental disability. Decerebration following injury sustained after the age of thirty-five is almost invariably followed by severe mental disability.

It was clear that however accurate these indices of long-term outcome are as an overall guide, they do not take account of individual variability. The prerequisite of accurate long-term prediction in the individual case would seem to be a detailed knowledge of the residual syndromes of mental and neurophysical disability which persist after severe acceleration brain injury. The recognition of these in convalescence, their degree, and the individual's response to them can then be examined against the general guide given by these predictive criteria. When progress is out of keeping, an explanation will be sought in the individual's constitutional intelligence or personality, focal ischaemic brain lesions superimposed upon lesser degrees of overall mechanical damage, the separate problems of epilepsy, cranial nerve injury and psychiatric illness precipitated but not to be expected in the majority, and finally simulation for gain.

This study has been concerned with the severest accidental acceleration head injuries. The most striking fact that emerges is how relatively uncommonly severe physical disability persists in the long-term, and how even incapacitating mental disability usually only persists with any frequency amongst the most severely injured. On the other hand, there was a small proportion of patients who, protected by their youth and modern techniques of resuscitation, survived such devastating brain damage that only the most insensitive would regard their survival as other than inhumane.

Two points follow from these observations. It is clear that for the majority of patients who sustain these severe head injuries almost every therapeutic effort will be worthwhile, since, in general, the outlook for at least acceptable or tolerable domestic, social and occupational rehabilitation is good. This is particularly the case in the young. In contrast, it is also very clear that every effort should continue to be made by those whose responsibility is the care of patients immediately after injury to identify, at the earliest stage, those who will survive only in vegetative or analogous states, or who will be so hideously disabled that their lives would be no more than an overwhelming burden to their relatives and the community.

It was impressed upon all who worked in this study and made contact with the patients or relatives that even for those whose recovery had been excellent the experience had been terrifying and disastrous. Most had suffered many weeks or months of misery, apprehensive of the significance of their amnesia, of continuing forgetfulness, defective concentration, imbalance and positional vertigo. Where there was any serious degree of personality change, however transient, the distress this caused the relatives was intense. It was not evident from this retrospective study what specific effects rehabilitative procedures had had nor what more appropriate provision might have been made. It did, however, seem that physiotherapists and nursing and medical staff in contact with the patients in hospital and in convalescence generally made an accurate assessment of the appropriate time for physical rehabilitation. In contrast, there appeared to have been an underestimate of the degree to which the patients and their relatives had been all but overwhelmed by the distressing effects of impaired intellectual function and personality change, even when these were relatively short-lived. Since the prognosis was at least acceptable in the majority of cases ultimately, even when serious mental disability was prolonged for 2 years or more, it would seem that greater efforts might justifiably be expended in order to provide closer and more skilled continuity of psychotherapeutic support and reassurance. On the evidence of this study such a provision would be best and most economically made by training of a small proportion of social workers as specialists in the needs and care of the head-injured and their families.

Finally, this study was designed on epidemiological lines to assess the long-term outcome of an equivalent of a random sample of severely head-injured patients from a clearly defined population of 7000 consecutive patients admitted to one regional accident service. This suggests that it may be possible to make some generalisations based on the results which might apply to the population at large.

It was noted by Field (1976) that, although each year the total number of patients admitted to hospital after head injury in England and Wales had varied from year to year, probably reflecting changing attitudes to the admission of the least severely injured, there had been a relatively constant 7000–8000 patients who had remained in hospital for 2 weeks or more before discharge or death. In other words there had been little change in the numbers of severely injured. These represent 6 per cent of an average 120 000 total number admitted to hospital after head injuries in England and Wales annually between 1962 and 1972. It does not seem unreasonable therefore to make the assumption that these, say 7000 patients, are similar to the 469, that is 6 per cent of the total population admitted to the Radcliffe Infirmary, with a post-traumatic amnesia of a week or more, selected for this study. In table 14.1 are set out the numbers and proportions of those who were followed up

Table 14.1   Numbers and percentages of patients in consecutive series totally or severely and profoundly disabled or 'recovered' at intervals in subsequent 25 years

Grade of persisting disability	Time since injury			
	6 months	1 year	10 years	25 years
Survivors examined				
Totals	291	291	291	221(Estimated)
Totally disabled	14(5%)	8(3%)	17(6%)	13(6%)
Severely and profoundly disabled	91(31%)	83(29%)	61(21%)	46(21%)
'Recovered'	186(64%)	200(69%)	213(73%)	162(73%)
Died after discharge				
Totals	75	68	23	
Totally disabled	4(5%)	2(3%)	1(6%)	
Severely and profoundly disabled	23(31%)	19(28%)	5(21%)	
'Recovered'	48(64%)	47(69%)	17(73%)	
Died of 'immediate' effects of head injury				
Totally disabled	10	3		
Entire sample				
Totals	469	469	469	469
Totally disabled	28(6%)	13(3%)	18(4%)	13(3%)
Severely and profoundly disabled	114(25%)	102(21%)	66(14%)	46(10%)
'Recovered'	238(51%)	247(53%)	230(49%)	162(34%)

(Consecutive series total 469 patients (6%) of 7000 patients admitted after head injury to Radcliffe Infirmary Regional Accident Service between 1948 and 1962, comprising every patient surviving amnesic or unconscious one week or more, and including 291 survivors examined, 103 who died of the 'immediate' effects of the injury, and 75 who recovered sufficiently to be discharged from hospital but died before the follow-up study.)

in the present study and found to be totally, or seriously and profoundly, disabled mentally or physically by their central neural lesions. It has been assumed that the 75 others who were no longer alive at the time of the follow-up study and had recovered sufficiently to be discharged from hospital were disabled in similar proportions. There was no evidence from the less detailed information available about them that suggested otherwise. The 103 who did not recover sufficiently to leave hospital before they died of their head injuries, but were alive 6 months and 1 year or more later have also been included in the calculations in this table. From these figures estimates have been made in table 14.2 of the numbers similarly disabled annually and

Table 14.2   Estimated numbers in population of England and Wales totally or severely and profoundly disabled after head injury each year assuming similar proportions among 7000 head injured annually remaining in hospital 2 weeks or more (6% of 120000 admitted to hospital after head injury annually)

Grade of persisting disability	Time since injury			
	6 months	1 year	10 years	25 years
Totally disabled	420	210	280	210
Severely or profoundly disabled	1750	1500	980	700

surviving for the next 25 years. Adjustments have been made to take account of the life expectancy in the population and that found in this study. It has also been assumed that negligible numbers whose injuries resulted in post-traumatic amnesia lasting less than a week will remain severely disabled. The justification for this assumption is the observation that only six out of 82 patients in the present study whose present post-traumatic amnesia lasted less than 2 weeks remained severely disabled in the long-term.

If these estimates can be accepted then it may be seen that each year in this country about 200 people survive injuries which leave them totally disabled for the rest of their lives, that is bed- or chairbound, or ambulant only with assistance, demented or psychotic so that they remain entirely dependent upon others. Another 1600 or so are left less severely disabled; however, their physical or mental disabilities preclude or substantially limit normal social or domestic life, or gainful employment. If the numbers of patients whose disabilities preclude gainful employment or normal domestic or social life are extracted from this latter group of less severely disabled, and combined with those who remain totally disabled, 32, that is 7 per cent, were alive in this state at 1 year amongst the consecutive series of patients. Applying this figure to the 7000 annually whose injuries confine them to hospital in England and Wales for a fortnight or longer it may be estimated that 490 may be expected to remain permanently disabled to a similar extent after head injuries each

year in this country. This is a figure close to the 500 'lame brains' who remain
unemployable after head injuries estimated by London (1967) on the basis of
figures derived from the Birmingham Accident Hospital and the population it
served.

On the basis of the three survivors and their length of survival in states of
decerebrate dementia in the consecutive series, and the numbers surviving in
similar states in both consecutive and selected series, estimates have been
made in table 14.3 of the numbers in England and Wales surviving annually,

Table 14.3 Numbers surviving in states of dementia and decerebration

	Years survival			
	1 year	3 years	5 years	10 years
Number of patients in the consecutive series	1	1	1	0
Number of patients in the combined consecutive and selected series	14(100%)	6(43%)	4(29%)	?1(??5%)
Estimated annual numbers (0.6%) among 7000 remaining in hospital 2 weeks or more and surviving in population of England and Wales	42(100%)	18(43%)	12(29%)	?2(??5%)
Number of vegetative survivors of head injury (after Higashi et al., 1977)	16(100%)	6(37%)	2(13%)	0

The three patients in the consecutive series represent 0.6 per cent of a 'sample'
population of 7000 patients admitted to Radcliffe Infirmary after head injury between
1948 and 1962.

and their likely period of survival. It is appreciated that the numbers are small
and the estimates wholly tentative, but it is reassuring to note that they are in
keeping with the figures of Higashi, Sakata, Hatano, Abiko, Ihara, Katayama,
Wakuta, Okamura, Ueda, Zenke and Aoki (1977) in a study of survivors in
vegetative and analogous states from Japan. The estimated figures for survival at 3 years are also not too dissimilar though higher in the present study for
5-year survival. As they found, the likelihood of survival for 10 years or more
was negligible, although it is clear that the occasional case does rarely survive
as long or longer than this.

It is appreciated that in making these estimates several assumptions have
been made which cannot be tested. It is possible also that these figures are
today underestimates both of the numbers of severely disabled surviving in
the past decade and a half due to advances in resuscitative techniques, and of

those with post-traumatic amnesia lasting less than a week who may have been left with more disability than was suggested by the present study of severer injuries. With these qualifications the figures give some idea of the size and nature of the problem of long-term disability after accidental head injury in the community.

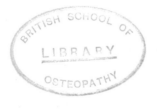

Appendix: Illustrative Cases

The following brief narrative summaries of case records of characteristic examples of each pattern of central neural and mental disability were dictated shortly after the patient had been seen. Their purpose was to provide a readily accessible overall picture of the patient and his disabilities. They therefore include only a small proportion of the data collected in each case by the author, neuropsychologist and social worker. The rest of the information is available in the detailed clinical records made out for every patient examined.

Case 1. Decerebrate Dementia: Vegetative
(D.B. age forty-six, Selected Series no. A63)

He was injured at the age of forty when his stock-car overturned in a race. There was no skull fracture, and it was recorded that there were 'no external injuries of any nature'. He was said to have been unconscious from the outset and when admitted to hospital locally was still unconscious and responding to pain, but there is no description of how. The pupils were unequal and neither reacted to light. Transferred within hours to Addenbrooke's Hospital, he was unrousable, with rigidity of the right more than the left limbs. At $2\frac{1}{2}$ weeks he remained with decerebrate extension of all limbs, developing opisthotonos in response to pain. A tracheostomy was made at 3 weeks. At 1 month spontaneous movements of the right arm were recorded. He remained decerebrate at the time of his transfer to a local hospital 7 weeks after the accident. Reviewed at 1 year, his eyes were open and he appeared to be looking round but the movements of his eyes were disconjugate. His legs were in decerebrate extension and his arms flexed. There were grasp reflexes on both sides. At 3 years his condition was the same and he remained mute, his eyes open but not certainly following, and there was no response apart from an increase in decerebrate tone to painful stimulation. There was extensive soft tissue peri-articular calcification. He seemed to sleep and wake and his general physical condition remained healthy due to the nursing attention he received. His spinal fluid at $2\frac{1}{2}$ weeks was clear and at normal pressure. An air encephalogram at 6 weeks revealed moderate ventricular dilatation, including the third ventricle, without evidence of obstruction.

Examined 5 years after his injury, his condition was unchanged except for the fact that entropion had resulted in corneal ulceration and blepharospasm of such a degree that it was not possible to examine his optic fundi. He was mute and unresponsive to the spoken word, responding to pain only by an increase in decerebrate tone, his arms flexing, his legs extending and his blepharospasm more marked. At rest increased muscle tone varied, according to the nurses, from one side to the other on different days. Sternal pressure caused the eyes to open and jerking movements without fixation were then briefly seen. He made occasional chewing movements spontaneously, but was tube-fed. There were brisk jaw, snout and palmomental reflexes. There was less decerebrate tone evoked by a pin in his left limbs than in his right. There was a periodic increase in his respiratory rate followed by relative apnoea. His tracheostomy was still patent. He had lost all his body hair apart from his beard within a few weeks 6 months earlier. His fingers were clubbed but his general physical condition was good and there were no pressure sores.

Case 2. Decerebrate Dementia
(E.P. age nineteen, Selected Series no. A53)

She was a back-seat passenger at the age of ten in a car which crashed head-on into a bus, killing the two front-seat occupants. There was no skull fracture and no note available to indicate the site of head impact. There is no account of her immediate state. Admitted locally she was deeply unconscious, her breathing stertorous, the right pupil fixed and dilated, and having 'occasional convulsions with rigidity between', presumably describing decerebrate attacks. Within an hour she was 'deeper' and the left pupil dilated so burr holes were made under local anaesthesia and 'some surface bleeding' was evacuated. The brain was described as 'bulging' after removal of these clots. Post-operatively she appeared to improve and then became 'deeper' again. The burr holes were reopened, bilateral subtemporal craniectomy decompressions made, and pulped temporal poles evacuated. Post-operatively the left pupil became smaller and there was an obvious right hemiplegia. She required ventilating and was transfused, and treated with steroids and diuretics. At 2 days her condition was unchanged and a tracheostomy was made. Transferred to the local neurosurgical unit at 10 days she remained deeply unconscious, the pupillary signs were unchanged, there was a left facial weakness, spontaneous movement of the left hand, and both her legs and right arm were in tonic extension. Her condition remained unchanged until her transfer back to the local hospital at 3 months. By 6 months she was taking fluids from a spoon and was responding by occasional smiles or by moving her eyes to her parent's voice. At 8 months she was examined by a paediatric neurologist and found to have optic atrophy, ocular deviation to the right with only occasional movements of the left eye laterally, a complete right third nerve palsy and a sluggish left pupillary response to light. There was a right-sided facial weakness, constant teeth grinding, tonic flexion of the neck and a spastic tetraplegia in flexion. The right leg was internally rotated and the left externally rotated, she was 'moving all her limbs to handling', and her right leg extended to altered head positioning and startle. Transferred to Addenbrooke's at 1 year there was 'no certain response to the external environment', but she 'roused' to noise and 'stirred' when handled. There was no reaction to menace but movements of her eyes suggested following responses, both discs were pale, the left more than the right, there was a right third nerve palsy, the left pupillary response was sluggish to light, the face was symmetrical, she was swallowing and her spastic tetraplegia was unchanged. Some spontaneous movement occurred in all limbs which also responded by reflex withdrawal to pain, more briskly on the right. Lumbar puncture at 12 days showed clear fluid, pressure at 200 and at 3 weeks the pressure was 120. Bilateral carotid angiograms at 12 days revealed poor filling suggesting raised intracranial pressure, but were otherwise normal. Air encephalography at 1 year demonstrated 'massive dilatation of the ventricular system, including the fourth, together with large basal cisterns and frontal sulci but no air over the vertex', indicating 'a complex external hydrocephalus', the arachnoid block being confirmed by isotope cisternography. She remained decerebrate, despite an atrio-ventricular shunt.

Examined at 4½ years after her injury it was evident that there had been some marginal alteration in the level of her responsiveness to stimulation, but it seemed that any response she made constituted merely a higher level reflex. She sat immobile in a chair making only an occasional spontaneous movement of her left wrist to scratch her nose. There were following responses of the eyes towards the sound and sight of her attendants. She responded by smiling to friendly words and by immobility and withdrawal to examination by a stranger. The highest level of neural function witnessed was laughter in response to the stimulus of her father chiding the dog. The physiotherapist who had treated her daily for the past 3 years claimed that in the last 2 she had begun to put out her tongue to his command. This could not be repeated by her parents' command during the examination, and it seemed likely that what actually occurred was that she responded by imitating his mimed gesture of tongue protrusion. When presented with a spoon filled with tea she opened her mouth in an apparently normal way which seemed possibly to be merely a complex bulbar reflex. The right disc was atrophic and the left less so. There was a sluggish consensual response of the left pupil to light but the right was fixed and dilated. The fields of vision of her left eye were evidently full, judging by her response to visual stimuli, but what vision remained in the right eye was uncertain. There was a complete right third nerve palsy, and incomplete abduction and adduction of the left eye. Corneal and facial sensation was normal but the face was strikingly impassive, and there was a slight right facial weakness. She responded to finger snapping, more briskly in the right than in the left ear. Teeth grinding was provoked by attempts to examine her. Her head and neck were in tonic flexion, as were all four limbs, left more than right. The only spontaneous limb movements seen were the stereotyped scratching movements made by her left arm. Reflex withdrawal was brisker in the left than the right limbs and it seemed that this was to some extent due to impaired perception of pain in the right limbs. There was a brisk snout and less easily elicited rooting reflex, the tendon jerks were pathologically brisk in the right arm and both plantar responses were extensor.

She was overweight, hirsute and doubly incontinent but her general condition was good and there were no bed sores.

The parents felt that $2\frac{1}{2}$ years after the injury she had begun for the first time clearly to show further improvement in her level of responsiveness. This was confirmed by the physiotherapist who had devoted so much of his time to her. It was at this time that she started laughing in response to appropriate stimuli, began to rub herself with her left arm, apparently purposefully and to make movements which suggested to him that she was trying to lift her right leg in response to his command. Over the next year he felt the range of her emotional expression, which had been limited to 'indifference and anguish' increased, she would put out her tongue, again apparently in response to his command, and she started to echo by some limited vocalisation his 'hallo'. She undoubtedly enjoyed her physiotheraphy and found pop music comforting. She had recently learned to move her tongue in her mouth to clear it of food preparatory to swallowing. There had been no certain improvement in her spastic tetraplegia, and the movement of the right leg considered by her parents and physiotherapist voluntary was clearly reflex.

This girl for practical purposes remained decerebrate. There had in the past 2 years been some definite increase in the range of her reflex responses which seemed largely still to be at bulbar level. There was no evidence of improvement following the insertion of the atrio-ventricular shunt a year after her injury. Her prolonged survival appeared due entirely to the devoted care, almost full-time, of both her parents and part-time enthusiastic physiotherapist and another voluntary helper. There seemed no reason to believe that she would have survived in different circumstances without such devoted care, or that she would survive should it cease to be available, but 6 years after the injury the illness of one and then both parents resulted in her admission to a hospital for the chronic sick where she remained, her condition unchanged 4 years later.

Case 3. Athetoid Pseudobulbar Syndrome with Frontolimbic Dementia
(F.B. age thirty-five, Consecutive Series no. 208)

He was flung from his motor-cycle at the age of twenty-three when he hit a dog. He was wearing a helmet. Linear right inferior temporal fractures running into the orbital roof together with right fronto-temporal abrasions and an orbital haematoma indicated a right fronto-lateral impact. He was described as 'unconscious when picked up'. Admitted to the Radcliffe Infirmary from the scene he was deeply unconscious without response to pain, his pupils were small possibly just reacting to light and there was slight respiratory obstruction. Shortly after admission he had three left-sided focal motor epileptic attacks. Within hours he was moving his arms in response to pain but not his legs, and generalised spasticity of the right more than the left limbs was noted. At one day he was opisthotonic, the decerebrate posture of his left arm and both legs being most marked, and his plantar responses were extensor. A tracheostomy was made and he was treated with hypothermia and chlorpromazine parenterally at a temperature of 91 °F (32.8 °C) for 5 days. There were no further decerebrate attacks during this procedure. At 1 week his left limbs remained in decerebrate extension. At 1 month he was opening his eyes and moving his left limbs purposefully, but these remained in extension, the right arm remained in flexion, the tendon jerks were brisker on the right than the left and both plantar responses were extensor. At 7 weeks his eyes were following, and he was moving his left but not his right limbs to command. At 9 weeks after closure of the tracheostomy, he was whispering in response to questions. At 11 weeks he was talking 'freely' but 'quietly'. He was then transferred to a local hospital. At 6 months there were brief records of the fact that he was sitting 'apathetically' and just walking with assistance. At 10 months his memory was poor, his speech slurred, his smile slow, and there was persisting impairment of ocular elevation and convergence, a dense right hemiparesis and he was obese. At 6 years he was continuing to have temper tantrums, there was a right-sided visual attention defect noted, and impairment of ocular elevation and convergence remained as did his right hemiparesis. Lumbar puncture at 1 day showed bloody fluid at a pressure of 190, at 1 week the pressure was 100 and the fluid yellow. Exploratory burr holes at 1 day revealed small bifrontal hygromata, and the left frontal horn was tapped producing bloody fluid. The brain was slack. An air encephalogram at 1 week, and a right carotid angiogram at 10 days suggested a space-occupying lesion of the corpus callosum. Air encephalography at 2 months demonstrated generalised dilatation of the lateral ventricles and basal cisterns. The PTA was assessed at 6 months.

Examined 12 years later he was evidently demented in that his mentation was profoundly slow, his anamnesis severely defective, and the content of his conversation strikingly limited. He was cheerful without being euphoric, and impressively disinhibited as judged by the swearing he indulged in during the interview. It seemed that the latter was also in some degree symptomatic of left temporal lobe injury since although he was without demonstrable dysphasia to routine nominal testing his repeated use of phrases like 'too true – yes mate' indicated severe expressive defect. His face was totally impassive and bilateral ptosis made him look sleepy and depressed. Changes of facial expression were slow to come and slow to go. His speech was profoundly slurred, apparently due to a combination of cerebellar ataxia and spasticity. There was a right-sided visual attention defect. Lateral conjugate gaze to the right was impaired and more so for the adducting than the abducting eye. The tongue protruded fully but repetitive movements were made very slowly. A right-sided facial weakness was associated with a dense right hemiparesis, the arm immobilised in flexion except at the wrist which was extended. There was marked extensor tone in both legs, on the right more than the left, and this was associated with pes cavus. All his movements were extremely slow, particularly his gait, which suggested extrapyramidal akinesia. The long pauses between moving from one leg to another, though with the aid of a walking stick, indicated considerable preservation of balance. He was just able to rise from a chair unaided and to take a few steps without help. Snout and jaw reflexes were brisk but tendon reflexes elsewhere were not notably brisk, though there was clonus of the right ankle and those in the left arm were less brisk than the right. Both plantar responses were extensor. A right-sided sensory inattention was present and associated with inability to discriminate two points on the right hand, defective joint position sense and impaired perception of pin on the right side including the face. General examination was unremarkable.

His recollection of the progress in his rehabilitation was poor and reliance had to be placed on details in hospital records and the independent account. He returned home to the care of his wife about 10 months after the injury and was then walking with the aid of a tripod, and soon with his wife's encouragement a stick. He was confined to the house by his disabilities and completely dependent on his wife. There was both urinary and faecal incontinence for the first year after his discharge from hospital but thereafter he had been continent. He was able in the following years to conceive 2 children. His continuing violent outbursts of temper in which he would belabour his small son, his sexual disinhibition together with the persisting dementia and physical disabilities proved too much for his wife. She and his son finally needed. psychotherapeutic support, and 6 years after his injury she divorced him. He had been resident in a home for the chronic sick since. The male nurse who accompanied him and who had known him well for 6 months described him as virtually confined to his chair but able to move with the aid of a stick a few steps. Apathy was not a notable feature in that he appeared to show spontaneous interest in his occupational therapy. On the other hand he had little interest in reading or the television and tended to drop off to sleep in front of the latter. A particular problem was his violent temper in which he would shake with fury and shout in a frightening high-pitched scream for several minutes at a time. This was provoked when he was crossed and also by minor irritations which related to disturbing his many obsessional rituals. Examples of these were the tantrums provoked by somebody failing to remove some dust or a cigarette end from close to him, nurses failing to do up the buttons of their white coats in front of him, the untidiness of other patients – three in particular for whom he had developed special dislikes – and of any disturbance in the ritual care with which he arranged the table cutlery. The nurses described him as very forgetful, never knowing where he had put things or asking repeatedly for things to be done for him which he had already asked and which had already been done.

There was no suggestion from the independent account of his ex-wife or the nurse who accompanied him of any deterioration in his intellectual functions or behaviour, or any worsening in his profound physical disabilities in the years since his injury.

Case 4. Severe Brainstem Cerebellar Syndrome and Frontolimbic Dementia

(C.C. age forty, Consecutive Series no. C30)

He drove his motor-cycle into a car at the age of twenty-one. He was not wearing a helmet. Left temporo-parietal fissured fractures and a sprung lamboid suture together with a left parieto-occipital haematoma indicate that the impact was left posterior parietal. There was no account of his immediate state. Admitted within a quarter of an hour from the scene to the Radcliffe Infirmary, he was unconscious, restless, his pupils contracting to light. He was moving spontaneously, but little in response to pain, his tendon jerks were symmetrical but the right plantar response was extensor. At 6 days he was deeply unconscious, his pupils fixed and dilated with decerebrate extensor tone of all four limbs together with periodic respiration. At 6 hours a left subtemporal craniectomy under local anaesthesia was made and an acute subdural haematoma evacuated. There were small lacerations of the left middle and inferior temporal convolutions and the brain here was 'very tight', but the right temporal lobe was slack. Post-operatively his pupils were smaller. At 2 days he remained decerebrate with decerebrate spasms more marked on the left than the right and a pyrexia of 103 °F (39.4 °C). He was cooled and treated with intravenous sucrose. His condition worsened and a tracheostomy was made. At 6 days he was moving his limbs in response to pain, his right pupil was reacting and there was less decerebrate tone but there was no further improvement so occipital burr holes under local anaesthesia were made and the craniectomy was re-explored. There were no clots but the right lateral ventricle was found to be small and only a few millilitres of CSF were removed. There was then increasing decerebration and at 9 days a left occipito-parietal craniectomy made under local anaesthesia exposed a swollen brain. Post-operatively he was flaccid. At 11 days he began making purposive brushing movements but was still having decerebrate spasms in response to pain, more marked on the right. At 1 month his eyes were open, there was constant chewing and in addition 'pill rolling' movements of the right hand; he was making purposeful movements in response to pain but there was still decerebrate tone and papilloedema. At 1½ months he was swallowing, and moving the right arm spontaneously and purposefully. At 2 months he was saying 'yes' and 'no', and the spasticity in his legs was less marked. At 4 months his eyes were following, there was a left third nerve palsy, he was smiling, able to put food into his mouth and standing with assistance. His face was expressionless, there was a right homonymous hemianopia and generalised spasticity. At 5 months he had two generalised convulsions, one beginning focally in the right arm. By 9 months he was saying an occasional word 'if surprised' and obeying promptly, looking at newspapers, smoking and walking with the assistance of one person. There was a persisting spastic tetraplegia, more marked on the right, and he tended to fall backwards standing unsupported. By 18 months he was continent. At 2½ years he was living at home, but remained without spontaneous speech, dysphasic, echolalic and bulaemic, but able to dress himself slowly. At 3 years his dementia and more particularly his violent tempers resulted in his confinement in a mental hospital. At 12 years while in the Radcliffe Infirmary for treatment of a urethral stricture, renal calculi and associated hypertension he was recorded as demented, dysphasic and still eating voraciously. Lumbar puncture at 2 days showed bloody fluid at a pressure of 240, and lumbar punctures were continued for 1½ weeks, the pressure being reduced by the removal of the fluid each time but still remaining in the region of 200 at 4 months. Post-traumatic dementia precluded the assessment of PTA.

Examined 20 years later he was genially demented. His manner was vague and he was distractable, almost without spontaneous speech and profoundly dysphasic in answering, grasping the instructions for the requirements of the examination occasionally quickly but more often only very tardily after repeated commands, and then tending to perseverate the information. His speech was slurred and his face strikingly impassive. Both optic discs were pale and the margins indistinct, suggesting secondary optic atrophy. There was a right homonymous hemianopia to fixation. The pupils were unequal and responded sluggishly to light. A brisk horizontal phasic nystagmus was present on lateral gaze to both sides, and on elevation there was vertical nystagmus. There was a slight right facial weakness and a slight left-sided probably conduction deafness. There was some weakness of both deltoids, more marked on the right, and weakness of hip flexion and dorsiflexion of the foot on the right. Slight spasticity was present in the right forearm pronators but he was generally hypotonic. All four limbs were ataxic, more so in the arms, and his gait was ataxic, wide-based, and right hemiparetic. He found it impossible to walk tandem fashion. The jaw jerk was present, the tendon reflexes brisk, but not excessively so, though brisker on the right, and the right plantar response was an indefinite extensor. Two point discrimination was accurate at 0.75 cm in the fingers of the right hand compared with 0.5 cm in the fingers of the left. General examination was remarkable only for the striae as evidence of the obesity before his recent weight loss due to rigid dieting. His blood pressure was within normal limits.

The patient's dementia and dysphasia precluded any account from him of his physical and intellectual disabilities since the injury. It was clear from the Radcliffe Infirmary and mental hospital records that the rehabilitation of his physical disabilities had progressed sufficiently by 2½ years for him to be fully mobile and self-sufficient in matters of toilet and dress, and to be discharged home. Thereafter, judging by his present moderate motor disabilities, further steady recovery took place though this is not recorded in detail. The principal disabling sequel of the injury was clearly the dementia and personality change. His frighteningly aggressive temper tantrums were the factor precipitating his admission to and permanent residence in a mental hospital, though according to the psychiatrist looking after him in the past 10 years the patient was in fact quite tractable. Although still liable to temper tantrums when teased he was never physically violent and retained a warm friendly personality which was a valuable aid in group therapy sessions in the chronic psychotic ward where he now lived. It seemed to some extent to be his parents' disinclination to burden themselves with their difficult son as much as his violent tempers which kept him resident in a mental hospital. It was not entirely clear from the information available but it seemed that he had his first fit about 3 years after the injury, and that these had recurred infrequently since such that they had never been a problem in management. Ten years ago he had been free of fits for 4 years until an attempt was made to discontinue his anticonvulsants. He then had further generalised convulsions and has remained on moderate doses of anticonvulsants since.

There is no suggestion from any of the sources available of any recent deterioration in intellectual functions or in his physical disabilities. Indeed it seems his vocabulary continues to increase over the years very slowly, and his unsteadiness and limb weakness together with his irritability has become less noticeable in the course of time.

Case 5. Mild Brainstem Cerebellar Syndrome with Traumatic Dysmnesia and Dysphasia
(C.B. age thirty-four, Consecutive Series no. S49)

She was wearing a riding hat when she fell from a horse at the age of sixteen. There was no account of scalp contusions and there were no fractures from which to deduce the site of impact to the head. There was no account of her immediate state but she was described as 'unconscious', and her condition remained unchanged during the 3 days she was in a local hospital. Transferred to the Radcliffe Infirmary at 3 days she was 'semi-conscious', groaning and moving her left more than her right limbs in response to pain, with a right facial weakness and a right pupil which was larger than the left. Tendon reflexes were brisker in the right limbs and both plantar responses were extensor. The paralysis in the right arm was recorded in the first few days as 'total'. At 6 days she was answering some questions and swallowing liquids. At 2 weeks she remained drowsy and disorientated but her right hemiparesis was recovering. At 3 weeks she was walking with assistance, her right hemiparesis was recorded as minimal but her speech was slurred and she was mildly dysphasic. There was impaired ocular convergence. She was euphoric. There was nystagmus on left more than right lateral gaze, ataxia of the left more than the right limbs, and her gait was unsteady. Reviewed at 6 weeks, and 3 and 6 months, these same signs were still present but less marked. The injury was complicated by a fracture of the right clavicle. Lumbar puncture at 4 days showed bloody fluid at a pressure of 160. The PTA extended for 3 weeks.

Examined 18 years later she seemed of above average intelligence, but vague and with a seriously defective memory as judged by her very imperfect anamnesis. There was a mild expressive dysphasia. Her face was slightly impassive. She was able to smell asafoetida rather less well with her right than the left nostril and she was unable to smell coffee. There was a mild inconstant left-sided external squint and she fixed preferentially with her right eye, but there was no definite ocular palsy or constantly demonstrable diplopia. She had a mild right facial weakness, and weakness of the right triceps and extensors of the fingers of the right hand. Repetitive movements were less well performed by the right than the left arm. There was a slight terminal ataxia of the right arm and leg. She found walking tandem fashion impossible and tended to lose her balance with her eyes shut. The tendon reflexes were brisker in the right limbs but both plantar responses were flexor. General examination was unremarkable.

She recalled as the principal sequel to her injury her imperfect memory for day-to-day events, slowness of thinking and the tardy manner in which she grasped what people said to her. She felt that associated with this there was a tendency to initiate but not develop conversation she was involved in, and she remained hesitant finding the right word. She had been aware that her balance had been poor since the injury, and that her right ankle would not dorsiflex as completely as the left, but she did not otherwise feel there were any persisting disabilities apart from her inconstant diplopia.

There was no evidence from her account or the account of her husband of any recent personality or intellectual deterioration, and no new physical disabilities had developed.

Case 6. Mild Brainstem Cerebellar Syndrome with Frontal Personality Change

(C.S. age thirty-four, Consecutive Series no. S118)

She was knocked off her bicycle by a car at the age of twenty. A right orbital haematoma and right frontal fissured fractures running into orbit and ethmoid indicate that the impact was right frontal. She was recorded as 'unconscious since the accident', becoming alert and responding to pain while in a local hospital 6 hours later. She developed a right hemiparesis on the day of her transfer. Admitted to the Radcliffe Infirmary 2 days after her accident she was unconscious, breathing stertorously and moving her left limbs more than her right, her tendon jerks were brisk and her plantars extensor. At 2 weeks she was mute apart from groaning, but moving in response to the spoken word. At $2\frac{1}{2}$ weeks she was speaking, her speech was slurred, there was a right external rectus weakness, impairment of ocular elevation and convergence, a right hemiparesis, and waxy flexibility of the limbs. On review at 3 months she was insightless and dysarthric, there was right-sided ataxia and the left plantar response was flexor but the right still extensor. These signs were still present but less marked at 6 and 18 months. Lumbar puncture at 4 days revealed pink fluid at a pressure of 190 and at 10 days it was clear, the pressure 100. Acute and convalescent stages were otherwise uncomplicated. The PTA was assessed at 3 weeks.

Examined 14 years later she appeared affectless and her thinking slow, but it was not clear whether this was obsessional or as a result of tardy intellectual function. She appeared lacking in full insight in that she was not aware of her minor persisting disabilities. Her intellectual functions appeared otherwise normal and she gave a well-documented account of her excellent memory for learning stage parts and poems since the accident, but she admitted to some absent-mindedness. Her face was strikingly impassive giving an impression of irritability or depression, the left pupil was larger than the right, there was a mild right facial weakness, and repetitive tongue movements were made very slowly. The tendon reflexes were brisker on the right than the left and the right plantar response was extensor. She found walking tandem fashion difficult though possible. General examination was unremarkable.

She could recall as her principal disabilities following discharge from hospital a tendency to sit without any inclination to do anything, which persisted for several months, a weakness of her right side which encouraged her to use her left and develop her normal ambidexterity, unsteadiness with inability to run for an indefinite time, the occasional hesitancy in finding the right word, and finally her inability to regain her previous level of scholarship at university reading mathematics. Her subsequent level of employment in the Meteorological Office evidently required above average intellectual abilities but it seemed certain that these were below those she previously had. She commented spontaneously on her tendency to be without interest in doing anything other than the most mundane of household chores and look after her children for whom, and also her husband, she noted she felt surprisingly little affection. This was confirmed by her husband.

There was no evidence either from the patient or her husband of any recent decline in intellectual functions or alteration in personality nor any progression in her mild persisting neural lesions.

Case 7. Dense Hemiparetic Pattern without Other Severe Neural Lesions

(R.J. age twenty-four, Consecutive Series S54)

He was knocked down by a lorry at the age of seven. Although abrasions of the head are mentioned there is no indication of the site of impact. Admitted locally within an hour he was unconscious with ocular elevation, dilated but reactive pupils, responding to pain, though it is not clear in what way, and there were occasional spontaneous extensor spasms on both sides together with ankle clonus and extensor plantar responses. He was bleeding from his mouth and right ear and there were moist sounds throughout his chest so that the impression was 'suffocation from blood'. At 24 hours he was in decerebrate extension with slight opisthotonus, and at 48 hours there were multiple retinal haemorrhages. At 2 days he was 'lighter', but again it is not clear how, with an obvious left hemiparesis but spasticity of all four limbs. At 3 weeks his eyes were open, he cried and smiled and was swallowing but he was still incontinent. At 1 month he was answering 'yes' and 'no', his speech was palatal and he was obeying commands. The right leg was still in decerebrate extension and there was a profound left hemiparesis with tendon jerks brisker on the left than the right, and both plantar responses were still extensor. At 6 weeks there was little improvement still in his left arm and leg, and he was transferred. Admitted to the Radcliffe Infirmary at 6 weeks he was dysarthric, with a spastic left hemiparesis and a spastic paresis of the right leg and ataxia of the right arm. At 8 weeks the left hemiparesis was improving slightly. Reviewed at 5 months he had returned to school and it appeared that he had forgotten how to read and write though his mother claimed there had been no behavioural changes. The spastic left hemiparesis and spastic right leg were still in evidence, but less marked, and his plantar responses were still extensor. At 1 and 2 years these signs were still present but again less marked. Lumbar puncture at 2 days was bloody, the pressure not recorded. Air encephalography at 2 months showed very slight asymmetrical dilatation. The acute stage was complicated by an aspiration pneumonia. The PTA does not appear to have been formally assessed but in retrospect extended for 6 weeks.

Examined 17 years later he appeared of average intelligence, tense and without any obvious defect in his memory functions as judged by his anamnesis. Although there was no demonstrable dysphasia his reading was laboured, even monosyllables being incorrectly pronounced at the first attempt. His writing was of poor quality but there was no definite dysgraphia. His face was not notably impassive but he had a moderate pseudobulbar dysarthria and his voice was palatal, and repetitive tongue movements were slowly and poorly performed. The left optic disc was atrophic, but it was not possible to demonstrate any field defect to a 5-mm red object. Visual acuity was N5 reading type in both eyes uncorrected. There was a mild left facial weakness. The left limbs were smaller than the right and spastic, and there were flexion contractures at the elbow, wrist and ankle. There was moderate weakness of flexors and abductors of the left hand, reasonable preservation of power of extension of the fingers but a total loss of movement of extension of the wrist, power proximally in the left arm was excellent. There was a moderate pyramidal weakness of the left leg and bilateral pes cavus. All the tendon reflexes were pathologically brisk, more so on the left, and the left plantar response was more briskly extensor than the right. There were brisk jaw and snout reflexes. General examination was unremarkable.

The patient's account of his disabilities following the injury were somewhat limited and reliance had to be placed on his mother's account. It seems that he returned to school whilst still virtually chairbound at about 5 months and as a result of this contact with his fellows again he was imbued with an urge to rehabilitate himself so that by the end of the year he was mobile on his own again. He had been aware of great difficulty learning anything from books since the injury when previously his scholastic level had been adequate if not brilliant. Despite this he has trained in the practice and theory of first aid for the St John's Ambulance Brigade and is an auxillary part-time nurse. Although he still has a dense residual left hemiplegia and moderate dysarthria he appears to have managed relatively heavy labouring jobs at different times in recent years. It seems likely that his physical disabilities have served to cut himself off from his fellows so that his main social contact outside the confines of his first aid work is with his mother.

There is no suggestion either from his or his mother's account of any recent personality or intellectual deterioration or any increase in his physical disabilities. Indeed the reverse in that in the last year slow improvement in his mobility has continued and for the first time he took himself abroad on holiday and alone.

Case 8. Mild Hemiparetic Pattern of Neural Lesions with Dysmnesic Inadequacy
(J.R. age fifty-nine, Consecutive Series S8)

She was thirty-nine when the car driven by her husband drove into the back of a lorry parked without lights. Lacerations of the left side of her face, ear, chest and hand, and dislocation of the left maxilla suggest that the main impact was to the left side of her head. There was no account of her immediate state. She was admitted within half an hour to the Radcliffe Infirmary and was then unconscious, moving in response to pain, her eyes deviated to the left, her jerks equal and her plantar responses recorded as flexor. Within hours she became hypotensive. She was transfused and was then talking. At 1 day she was answering occasional questions and obeying some commands, the tendon reflexes were brisker in the right limbs and both plantar responses were flexor. At 5 days she was confused, there was slight dysphasia, and a slight right-sided hemiparesis with an indefinite right extensor plantar response. At 12 days she was orientated. At 3 weeks she still had a mild right hemiparesis and was transferred to a nursing home. Reviewed at 5 months she was complaining of giddiness and was slightly dysphasic, there was left-sided deafness, and the mild right-sided hemiparesis with brisker right-sided jerks was still present. At 1 year she complained of tiring easily and of poor concentration, and her dysphasia was still apparent. There was now only an asymmetry of the tendon reflexes which were brisker in the right arm as evidence of the hemiparesis she had. The injury was complicated by fractures of the left and right mandibles which were treated by splinting under general anaesthesia within hours of the injury. There were also fractures of the transverse processes of the fifth and sixth cervical vertebrae. Lumbar puncture at 4 days showed bloody fluid at a pressure of 100. The PTA was assessed at 9 days.

Examined 19 years later she seemed of above average intelligence, and without memory defect as judged by her anamnesis, though she claimed that her memory for day-to-day events had been mildly defective since the injury. There was no formal dysphasia either in conversation or on naming common objects, though she was aware she was occasionally hesitant for a word still. Her face was slightly immobile and asymmetrical by virtue of scarring. There was a slight left perceptive deafness which was a sequel of the injury. Slight weakness in pyramidal distribution was demonstrable in the right arm and repetitive movements of the right arm and hand were less well performed than with the left. Tendon reflexes were brisker in the right limbs and the right plantar response was an indefinite extensor. General examination was notable only for her blood pressure of 200/110 without evidence of retinopathy.

She recalled as her principal disabilities following the injury forgetfulness for day-to-day events and slowness of thought, and although this improved in the first year they appeared to have made her unwilling to leave the house alone and avoid shopping by herself for even longer. She did not recall any specific weakness of the limbs, only that she had been easily tired. These symptoms were marked for at least 2 years and still persist in some degree. She claimed not to have had any tendency to worry over trifles before the injury but that she had been a constant worrier since. Previously sociable her dysphasia and possibly her mild facial disfigurement made her unwilling to meet other people and she had tended to remain less sociable. Before the accident she had given her husband secretarial help but afterwards she had given up typing and had not worked since.

There is no suggestion from her account or that of her husband of any recent alteration in personality or intellectual functions, and there has been no increase in her very minor physical disabilities.

Case 9. Phobic Imbalance and Dysmnesic Inadequacy
(F.A. age seventy-seven, Consecutive Series S122)

He was knocked from his cycle at the age of sixty-three. A laceration of the left ear was the only indication of the site of head impact. He was smelling of alcohol when found lying by his bike on the road. He was admitted from the scene to the Radcliffe Infirmary and was then unconscious, 'rousing to pain', but his limbs flaccid. Within half an hour he was moving all his limbs spontaneously, the left more than the right, the tendon reflexes were brisker and the tone increased in the right more than the left limbs, and both plantar responses were extensor. At 5 days his blood urea was 120 mg per cent. At 1 week he said 'hello', and at that time it was noted that he had a left peripheral facial weakness. At 2 weeks he appeared to deteriorate and ceased to respond verbally, and this was associated with the development of acidotic respiration. At 2½ weeks he was talking again. He remained confused for 5 weeks. Reviewed at 6 months he was experiencing positional vertigo, his gait was noted to be 'stiff' and 'unsteady', there was a left facial weakness but he had begun gardening again. At 10 and 15 months these same signs were still present but less marked. The injury was complicated by a fracture of the left scapula and several ribs. Lumbar puncture at 1 day showed bloody fluid at a pressure of 110. The PTA was assessed at 2 months.

Examined 14 years later there was no evidence of the head injury he had sustained. It appeared from his wife's account that some time after his return home from hospital he was very forgetful and unsteady on his feet and his speech was slurred. Despite steady improvement he remained fearful of leaving the house alone to cross a road and would have a 'shaking fit' at the thought of having to do so. He later managed to take himself for walks, but he never returned to work and spent most of his time pottering about his garden. He seemed to lose the confidence to organise his daily life and became very dependent on his wife, which he had not been before.

There was no suggestion from his wife's account that there had been any alteration in his intellectual functions or personality as he grew older.

Case 10. Traumatic Depression
(J.C. age fifty, Consecutive Series S207)

He was knocked down by a motor cycle at the age of thirty-seven. There were fractures of both mandibular rami and contusions of the left orbit and left parietal region suggesting uncertainly that the primary impact of the head was left fronto-lateral. He was smelling of alcohol and his pupils were described as dilated before the doctor gave him morphine. Admitted to the Radcliffe Infirmary within an hour he was drowsy, confused, blaspheming and shouting 'leave me alone'. All limbs were moving spontaneously and to pain but he did not obey commands, his eye movements were disconjugate, his tendon reflexes equal and the plantar responses flexor. He improved progressively to full orientation at 2 weeks. Reviewed at 2 months he complained that he was a 'bag of nerves'. At 2 and 2½ years he appeared introspective and depressed but there were no other signs of injury. Lumbar puncture at 5 days revealed yellow fluid at a pressure of 80. The injury was complicated by a fracture of the left tibia. The PTA was assessed at 2 weeks.

Examined 12 years later he appeared tense, introspective to a degree that might be described as preoccupied, and of average intelligence. As judged by his detailed anamnesis there was no defect of memory functions. There were facial tics and a mild right facial weakness but no other abnormal neural signs. General examination was unremarkable.

He recalled as the principal sequel of the injury phobic and depressive symptoms which at one time confined him to the house and disabled him completely for about 2 years and intermittently thereafter. He required inpatient psychiatric treatment and was still taking a tricyclic antidepressant regularly as he had been for the past 7 years.

There was no suggestion from the patient or his wife of any recent deterioration in his intellectual functions or personality and he had not developed any new physical disabilities. Indeed according to his wife it is only in the past 3 years since he had taken a less demanding job as a school caretaker and handyman that his neurotic illness ceased to disable him so completely.

References

Adams, H., and Graham, D. I. (1972). The relationship between ventricular fluid pressure and the neuropathology of raised intracranial pressure. In: Brock, M. and Dietz, H., eds *Intracranial Pressure*. Berlin, pp. 250 ff.

Akerlund, E. (1959). The late prognosis in severe head injuries. *Acta clin. scand.*, **117**, 275–7

Albert, M. L., Feldman, R. G. and Willis, A. L. (1974). The subcortical dementia of progressive supranuclear palsy. *J. Neurol. Neurosurg. Psychiat.*, **37**, 121–30

Alquié, A. (1865). Étude clinique et expérimentale de la commotion traumatique ou ébranlement de l'encéphale. *Gaz. méd. Paris*, **36**, 226–30, 254–6, 314–9, 382–5, 396–8, 463–6, 500–4 (Third Series)

Andrew, J. and Nathan, P. W. (1965). The cerebral control of micturition. *Proc. R. Soc. Med.*, **58**, 553–5

Bard, P. and Mountcastle, V. B. (1948). Some forebrain mechanisms involved in expression of rage with special reference to suppression of angry behavior. Association for Research in Nervous and Mental Disease. Research Publications, **27**, 362–404 (*The Frontal Lobes*. Baltimore, Williams and Wilkins, 1948)

Baughan, B. (1973). Program GUMMA. The universal multivariate analyser. London, Institute of Education Computing Centre

Behrman, S. (1975). Hostility to kith and kin. *Br. med. J.*, **2**, 538–9

Bevilacqua, G. and Fornaciari, G. (1975). Clinico-pathological correlations in a case of post traumatic pan-hypopituitarism. *Acta neuropath.*, **31**, 171–7

Black, P., Jefferies, J. J., Blumer, D., Wellner, A. and Walker, A. E. (1969). The post-traumatic syndrome in children. Characteristics and incidence. In: Walker, A. E., Caveness, W. F. and Critchley, M. (eds), *The Late Effects of Head Injury*. Springfield, Ill., Charles C. Thomas, pp. 142–9

Bokonjic, N., and Buchthal, F. (1961). Post anoxic unconsciousness as related to clinical and EEG recovery in stagnant anoxia and carbon monoxide poisoning. In: Meyer, J. S., and Gastaut, H. (eds), *Cerebral Anoxia and the Electroencephalogram*. Springfield, Ill., Charles C. Thomas, pp. 118–27

Boller, F. C., Albert, M. L., Le May, M., and Kertesz, A. (1972). Enlargement of the Sylvian aqueduct: a sequel of head injuries. *J. Neurol. Neurosurg. Psychiat.*, **35**, 463–7

Bond, M. R. (1975). Assessment of the psychosocial outcome after severe head injury. In: Porter, R., and Fitzsimons, D. W. (eds), *Outcome of Severe Damage to the Central Nervous System*. Amsterdam, Elsevier, Excerpta Medica (Ciba Foundation Symposium 34, New Series), pp. 141–57

Bowman, K. M., and Blau, A. (1960). Psychotic states following head and brain injury in adults and children. In: Brock, S. (ed.), *Injuries of the Brain and Spinal Cord and their Coverings*, 4th edn, London, Cassell, pp. 360–409

Breasted, H. J. (1930). *The Edwin Smith Surgical Papyrus.* Chicago, Ill., University of Chicago Press, pp. 203–16

Brewis, M., Poskanzer, D. C., Rolland, C., and Miller, H. (1966). Neurological disease in an English city. *Acta neurol. scand.*, **42**, Suppl. 24

Brierley, J. B. (1971). The neuropathological sequelae of profound hypoxia. In: Brierley, J. B., and Meldrum, B. S. (eds), *Brain Hypoxia.* London, William Heinemann, pp. 147–51

Brierley, J. B., and Excell, B. J. (1966). The effects of profound systemic hypotension upon the brain of *M. rhesus*: physiological and pathological observations. *Brain*, **89**, 269–98

Brink, J. D., Garrett, A. L., Hale, W. R., Woo-Sam, J., and Nickel, V. L. (1970). Recovery of motor and intellectual function in children sustaining severe head injuries. *Devl Med. Child Neurol.*, **12**, 565–71

Broca, P. (1878). Anatomie comparée des circonvolusions cérébrales. *Rev. anthropol.*, **1**, 385–498 (Series 3)

Bruckner, F. E., and Randle, A. P. H. (1972). Return to work after severe head injuries. *Rheumatol. phys. Med.*, **11**, 344–8

Burzaco, J. A., and Gutiérrez Gomez, D. (1968). Trastorno de conducta postencefalitico (su tratamiento por cirugia estereotáxica). *Arch. Neurobiol., Madrid*, **31**, 69–77

Cairns, H., Oldfield, R. C., Pennybacker, J. B., and Whitteridge, D. (1941). Akinetic mutism with an epidermoid cyst of the 3rd ventricle. *Brain*, **64**, 273–90

Carlsson, C.-A., Essen, C. von, and Löfgren, J. (1968). Factors affecting the clinical course of patients with severe head injuries. Part 1: Influence of biological factors. Part 2: Significance of posttraumatic coma. *J. Neurosurg.*, **29**, 242–8, 248–51

Caveness, W. F. (1963). Onset and cessation of fits following craniocerebral trauma. *J. Neurosurg.*, **20**, 570–83

Caviness, V. S. (1969). Epilepsy: a late effect of head injury. In: Walker, A. E., Caveness, W. F., and Critchley, M. (eds), *The Late Effects of Head Injury.* Springfield, Ill., Charles C. Thomas, pp. 193–200

Ciompi, L. (1972). Long term follow up study of the process of aging in patients with former brain injury. *Arbeitsmed. Sozialmed. Arbeitshyg.*, **7**, 191–3

Clark, J. M. (1974). Distribution of microglial clusters in the brain after head injury. *J. Neurol. Neurosurg. Psychiat.*, **37**, 463–74

Claude, H., and Cuel, J. (1939). Démence pré-sénile post-traumatique après fracture du crâne; considérations medico-légales. *Ann. Méd. légale*, **19**, 173–84

Cohadon, F., Hubert, L. M., and Richter, E. (1972). The process of rehabilitation in patients with severe cranial injury. Results of a series of 190 injured patients. Frequency, nature and final consequences of the sequels. *Bordeaux Méd.*, **5**, 2387–96

Cohadon, F. Hubert, L. M., and Richter, E. (1972). Fréquence des séquelles et problèmes qu'elles posent durant le processus de réhabilitation. *Neurochirurgie*, **18**, 209–17 (Suppl. 2)

Corsellis, J. A. N. (1962). *Mental Illness and the Ageing Brain.* Oxford, Oxford University Press

Corsellis, J. A. N. (1975). Unpublished paper given at a meeting of the Neurology Section of the Royal Society of Medicine, February 1975

Corsellis, J. A. N. (1976). Ageing and the dementias. In: Blackwood, W., and Corsellis, J. A. N. (eds), *Greenfield's Neuropathology*, 3rd edn, London, Edward Arnold, pp. 796–848

Corsellis, J. A. N. (1976). *Lancet*, **i**, 401–2

Corsellis, J. A. N., and Brierley, J. B. (1959). Observations on the pathology of insidious dementia following head injury. *J. ment. Sci.*, **105**, 714–20

Corsellis, J. A. N., and Roberts, A. H. (1975). Unpublished data

Corsellis, J. A. N., Bruton, C. J., and Freeman-Browne, D. (1973). The aftermath of boxing. *Psychol. Med.*, **3**, 270–303

Courville, C. B. (1942). Coup-contrecoup mechanism of cranio-cerebral injuries. Some observations. *Arch. Surg., Chicago*, **45**, 19–43

Courville, C. B. (1950). The mechanism of coup-contrecoup injuries of the brain. A critical review of recent experimental studies in the light of clinical observations. *Bull. Los Angeles neurol. Soc.*, **15**, 72–86

Courville, C. B. (1958). Traumatic lesions of the tempral lobe. In: Baldwin, M., and Bailey, P. (eds). *Temporal Lobe Epilepsy*. Springfield, Ill. Charles C. Thomas, pp. 220–239

Crompton, M. R. (1970). Visual lesions in closed head injury. *Brain*, **93**, 785–92

Daghighian, I. (1973). The aging of persons with past cranial injury. (Retrospective study of 88 patients hospitalized in a psychiatric service.) *Schweiz. Arch. Neurol. Neurochir. Psychiat.*, **112**, 399–447

Davison, K., and Bagley, C. R. (1969). Schizophrenia-like psychoses associated with organic disorders of the central nervous system: a review of the literature. In: Herrington, R. N. (ed.), *Current Problems in Neuropsychiatry. (British Journal of Psychiatry* Special Publication No. 4). Ashford, Kent, Headley Brothers Ltd, pp. 113–84

Dawson, R. E., Webster, J. E., and Gurdjian, E. S. (1951). Serial electroencephalography in acute head injuries. *J. Neurosurg.*, **8**, 613–30

Deruty, R., Dumas, R., Dechaume, J.-P., Lecuire, J., Girard, R., and Bourret, J. (1970). Study of the remote future of prolonged posttraumatic comas. *Ann. Méd. phys.*, **13**, 3–20

Dolce, G., and Fromm, H. (1972). An experimental model of the apallic syndrome. *Scand. J. Rehabil. Med.*, **4**, 39–43

Elithorne, A., Kerr, M., and Jones, D. (1963). A binary perceptual maze. *Am. J. Psychol.* **76**, 506–8

Elsässer, G., and Grünewald, H.-W. (1953). Schizophrenie oder schizophrenieähnliche Psychosen bei Hirntraumatikern. *Arch. Psychiat.*, **190**, 134–49

Fahy, T. J., Irving, M. H., and Millac, P. (1967). Severe head injuries. A six-year follow-up. *Lancet*, **ii**, 475–9

Fallopius, G. (1584). *Opera omnia*. Frankfurt, Andreae Wecheli, pp. 692 ff.

Field, J. H. (1976). *Epidemiology of Head Injuries in England and Wales*. London, HMSO

Fishgold, H., and Mathis, P. (1959). Obnubliations, comas et stupeurs. *Electroenceph. clin. Neurophysiol.*, Suppl. 11, pp. 81 ff.

Flach, J., and Malmros, R. (1972). A long term follow up study of children with severe head injury. *Scand. J. Rehabil. Med.*, **4**, 9–15

Foltz, E. L., and Ward, A. A. (1956). Communicating hydrocephalus from subarachnoid bleeding. *J. Neurosurg.*, **13**, 546–66

Freytag, E. (1963). Autopsy findings in head injuries from blunt forces. Statistical evaluation of 1367 cases. *Arch. Pathol.*, **75**, 402–13

Frowein, R. A., Haar, auf der K., Terhaag, T., Kinzel, W., and Wieck, H. H. (1968). Capacity for work and the degeneration syndrome after cerebral trauma with prolonged unconsciousness. 100 clinical investigations and 38 psychologically tested cases among adults and children. *Monats. Unfallheil. Versicherungsmed.*, **71**, 233–49

Gammie, J. W. (1977). Personal communication

Gerstenbrand, F. (1967). *Das traumatische apallische Syndrom. Klinik, Morphologie, Pathophysiologie und Behandlung.* Vienna, Springer Verlag

Gerstenbrand, F., Lucking, C. H., Peters, G., and Rothemund, E. (1970). Cerebellar symptoms as sequelae of traumatic lesions of upper brain stem and cerebellum. *Int. J. Neurol.*, **7**, 271–82

Gibson, J. M. C. (1960). Multiple injuries: the management of the patient with a fractured femur and a head injury. *J. Bone Jt Surg.*, **42B**, 425–31

Glenn, J. N., Miner, M. E., and Peltier, L. F. (1973). The treatment of fractures of the femur in patients with head injuries. *J. Trauma*, **13**, 958–61

Goldman, K. P., and Jacobs, A. (1960). Anterior and posterior pituitary failure after head injury. *Br. med. J.*, **4**, 1924–6

Goldsmith, W. (1970). Biomechanics of head injury. In: Fung, Y. C., Pernone, N., and Anliker, M. (eds), *Biomechanics, its Foundations and Objectives*, Englewood Cliffs, N.J., Prentice-Hall, pp. 585–634

Gordon, E. (1972). Controlled ventilation in the management of patients with severe head injuries. *Scand. J. Rehabil. Med.*, **4**, 21–3

Graham, D. I., and Adams, J. H. (1971a). Ischaemic brain damage in fatal head injuries. *Lancet*, **i**, 265–6

Graham, D. I., and Adams, J. H. (1971b). Ischaemic brain damage in fatal head injuries. In: Brierley, J. B., and Meldrum, B. S. (eds), *Brain Hypoxia*. London, Heinemann Medical (Clinics in Developmental Medicine **39/40**), pp. 34–40

Granholm, L., and Svengaard, N. (1972). Hydrocephalus following traumatic head injuries. *Scand. J. Rehabil. Med.*, **4**, 31–4

Grima. (1766). Sur les contre-coups dans les lesions de la tête. In: *Mémoires sur les sujets proposés pour les prix de l'Academie Royale de Chirurgie*, tome quatrième, premier partie. Chez Ménard et Desenne, Fils, Libraires, 1819, pp. 207–26

Grob, U., and Ketz, E. (1974). Posttraumatic epilepsy after depressed fracture of the skull. *Schweiz. med. Wochenschr.*, **104**, 209–12

Gronwall, D., and Wrightson, P. (1974). Delayed recovery of intellectual function after minor head injury. *Lancet*, **ii**, 605–9

Gurdjian, E. S., and Webster, J. E. (1958). *Head Injuries: Mechanisms, Diagnosis and Management.* Boston and Toronto, Little Brown & Co.

Gurdjian, E. S., Webster, J. E., and Arnkoff, H. (1943). Acute craniocerebral trauma. Surgical and pathologic considerations based upon 151 consecutive autopsies. *Surgery*, **13**, 333–53

Gurdjian, E. S., Webster, J. E., and Lissner, H. R. (1950). The mechanism of skull fracture. *J. Neurol.*, **7**, 106–14

Gutterman, P., and Shenkin, H. A. (1970). Prognostic features in recovery from traumatic decerebration. *J. Neurosurg.*, **32**, 330–5

Guttmann, Sir L. (1976). *Spinal Cord Injuries*, 2nd edn, Oxford, Blackwell

Hakim, S., and Adams, R. D. (1965). The special clinical problem of symptomatic hydrocephalus with normal cerebrospinal fluid pressure. Observations on cerebrospinal fluid hydrodynamics. *J. neurol. Sci.*, **2**, 307–27

Harrison, M., and Ozsohinoglu, C. (1972). Positional vertigo: aetiology and clinical significance. *Brain*, **95**, 369–72

Hassler, R., Dalle Ore, G., Dieckmann, G., Bricolo, A., and Dolce, G. (1969). Behavioral EEG arousal induced by stimulation of unspecific projection systems in a patient with post-traumatic apallic syndrome. *Electroenceph. clin. Neurophysiol.*, **27**, 306–10

Heilmann, K. M., Saffran, A., and Geschwind, N. (1971). Closed head trauma and aphasia. *J. Neurol. Neurosurg. Psychiat.*, **34**, 265–9

Heiskanen, O., and Kaste, M. (1974). Late prognosis of severe brain injury in children. *Devl Med. Child Neurol.*, **16**, 11–14

Heiskanen, O., and Sipponen, P. (1970). Prognosis of severe head injury. *Acta neurol. scand.*, **46**, 343–8

Hetherington, A. W., and Ranson, S. W. (1940). Hypothalamic lesions and adiposity in the rat. *Anat. Rec.*, **78**, 149–72

Higashi, K., Sakata, Y., Hatano, M., Abiko, S., Ihara, K., Katayama, S., Wakuta, Y., Okamura, T., Ueda, H., Zenke, M., and Aoki, H. (1977). Epidemiological studies on patients with a persistent vegetative state. *J. Neurol. Neurosurg. Psychiat.*, **40**, 876–85

Hillbom, E. (1951). Schizophrenia-like psychoses after brain trauma. *Acta psychiat. neurol. scand.*, Suppl. 60, 36–47

Hillbom, E. (1960). After effects of brain injuries. *Acta psychiat. neurol. scand.*, Suppl. 142

Hinoki, M. (1971). Equilibrium tests with adrenaline loading: their clinical value in the diagnosis of brain stem disorder as related to vertigo due to head injury. *Tokushima J. exptl Med.*, **18**, 1–14

Hirakawa, K., Hashizume, K., Nakamura, N., and Sano, K. (1971). Mechanical study on the traumatic optic nerve injury. *Neurol. med.-chir., Tokyo*, **11**, 34–45

Hoare, E. M. (1971). Platelet response in fat embolism and its relationship to petechiae. *Br. med. J.*, **2**, 689–90

Holbourn, A. H. S. (1943). Mechanics of head injuries. *Lancet*, **ii**, 438–41

Holbourn, A. H. S. (1944). The mechanics of trauma with special reference to herniation of cerebral tissue. *J. Neurosurg.*, **1**, 190–200

Holbourn, A. H. S. (1945). The mechanics of brain injuries. *Br. med. Bull.*, **3**, 147–9

Hollander, D. (1968). Atypical Alzheimer's disease. Unpublished dissertation for the Academic DPM, University of London

Hollander, D., and Strich, S. J. (1970). Atypical Alzheimer's disease with congophilic angiopathy presenting with dementia of acute onset. In: Wolstenholme, G. E., and O'Connor, M. (eds), *Alzheimer's Disease and*

Related Conditions. London, Churchill, pp. 103–35 (Ciba Foundation Symposium)

Hooper, R. S. (1951). Orbital complications of head injury. *Br. J. Surg.*, **39**, 126–38

Hooper, R. S., McGregor, J. M., and Nathan, P. W. (1945). Explosive rage following head injury. *J. mental Sci.*, **91**, 458–71

Hughes, B. J. (1964). The results of injury to special parts of the brain and skull. In: Rowbotham, G. R. (ed.), *Acute Injuries of the Head. Their Diagnosis, Treatment, Complications and Sequels*, 4th edn, Edinburgh and London, E. & S. Livingstone, pp. 408–33

Ingvar, D. H. (1975). Discussion following: Card, W. I. (1975). Development of a formal structure for clinical management decisions: a mathematical analysis. In: Porter, R., and Fitzsimons, D. W., eds. *Outcome of Severe Damage to the Central Nervous System.* Amsterdam, Elsevier, Excerpta Medica, p. 302 (Ciba Foundation Symposium **34**. New Series)

Jefferson, A. and Reilly, G. (1972). Fractures of the anterior cranial fossa. The selection of patients for dural repair. *Br. J. Surg.*, **59**, 585–92

Jellinger, K., and Seitelberger, F. (1970). Protracted post-traumatic encephalopathy. Pathology, pathogenesis and clinical implications. *J. neurol. Sci.*, **10**, 51–94

Jennett, W. B. (1962). *Epilepsy after Blunt Head Injuries.* London, Heinemann Medical

Jennett, W. B. (1969). Early traumatic epilepsy. *Lancet*, **i**, 1023–5

Jennett, W. B. (1970). Secondary ischaemic brain damage after head injury. *J. clin. Pathol.*, **4**, 172–5 (Suppl. 23)

Jennett, W. B. (1975). Epilepsy and acute traumatic intracranial haematoma. *Neurol. Neurosurg. Psychiat.*, **38**, 378–81

Jennett, W. B., and Lewin, W. (1960). Traumatic epilepsy after closed head injuries. *J. Neurol. Neurosurg. Psychiat.*, **23**, 295–301

Jennett, W. B., and Plum, F. (1972). Persistent vegetative state after brain damage. A syndrome in search of a name. *Lancet*, **i**, 734–7

Jennett, W. B., Miller, J. D., and Braakman, R. (1974). Epilepsy after non-missile depressed skull fracture. *J. Neurosurg.*, **41**, 208–16

Jennett, W. B., Teasdale, G. M., and Knill-Jones, R. P. (1975). Predicting outcome after head injury. *J. R. Coll. Physicians Lond.*, **9**, 231–7

Jennett, W. B., Teasdale, G., Galbraith, S., Pickard, J., Grant, H., Braakman, R., Avezaat, C., Maas, A., Minderhoud, J., Vecht, C. J., Heiden, J., Small, R., Caton, W., and Kurze, T. (1977). Severe head injuries in three countries. *J. Neurol. Neurosurg. Psychiat.*, **40**, 291–8

Johnson, T. N., Rosvold, H. E., and Mishkin, M. (1968). Projections from behaviourally-defined sectors of the prefrontal cortex to the basal ganglia, septum and diencephalon of the monkey. *Expl Neurol.*, **21**, 20–34

Kay, D. W. K., Beamish, P., and Roth, M. (1964). Old age mental disorders in Newcastle-upon-Tyne. *Br. J. Psychiat.*, **110**, 146–58

Kinzel, W. (1968). Die quantitative Abschätzung des psychischen Defektsyndroms nach Hirnkontusion. Dissertation, Erlängen

Kleist, K. (1922/1934). Das Stirnhirn (im engeren Sinn) und die ihm eigenen Störungen und Bewegungen . . . Antrieb, Handeln und Denken. In: Schjerning, O. von (ed.), *Handbuch der Ärtzlichen Erfahrungen im Welt-*

kriege 1914/1918. Band IV: Bonhoeffer, K. (ed.), *Geistes- und Nerven-krankheiten.* Leipzig, Johann Ambrosius Barth Verlag, p. 934

Kluver, H., and Bucy, P. C. (1939). Preliminary analysis of functions of the temporal lobes in monkeys. *Arch. Neurol. Psychiat., Chicago,* **42**, 979–1000

Kremer, M. (1944). Discussion on disorders of personality after head injury. *Proc. R. Soc. Med.,* **37**, 564–6

Kremer, M., Russell, W. R., and Smyth, G. E. (1947). A mid-brain syndrome following head injury. *J. Neurol. Neurosurg. Psychiat.,* **10**, 49–60

Kretschmer, E. (1940). Das apallische Syndrom. *Z. ges. Neurol. Psychiat.,* **169**, 576–9

Kretschmer, E. (1949). Cerebral orbital and diencephalic syndromes follow-ing fractures of the base of the skull. *Arch. Psychiat.,* **182**, 452–77

Lambooy, N., van der Zwan, A., and Fossen, A. (1965). End-results after long term unconsciousness due to head injury. *Psychiat. neurol. neurochir., Amsterdam,* **68**, 431–42

Lechner, H. (1958). Zur Deutung der Symptomatologie der temporalen Kontusionen. *Wien. klin. Wochenschr.,* **70**, 365–70

Lecuire, J. (1974). Long term evaluation of severe cranio-cerebral injuries with protracted coma. *Ann. Méd. Accidents Trafic,* **2**, 14–16

Lecuire, J., Deruty, R., Dechaume, J.-P., and Lapras, C. (1973). Present considerations on the remote course of severe head injuries with pro-tracted coma. *Neurochirurgie,* **19**, 271–7

Legg, N. J., Gupta, P. C., and Scott, D. F. (1973). Epilepsy following cerebral abscess. A clinical and EEG study of 70 patients. *Brain,* **96**, 259–68

Lehnhardt, E. (1974). Audiological characteristics of central deafness follow-ing head injuries. *Arch. Otolaryngol.,* **208**, 163–74

Lewin, W. (1965). Observations on prolonged unconsciousness after head injury. In: Cumings, J. N., and Kremer, M. (eds), *Biochemical Aspects of Neurological Disorders,* 2nd edn, Oxford, Blackwell, pp. 182 ff.

Lewin, W. (1966). *The Management of Head Injuries.* London, Baillière, Tindall & Cassell

Lewin, W. (1968a). Preliminary observations on external hydrocephalus after severe head injury. *Br. J. Surg.,* **55**, 747–51

Lewin, W. (1968b). Rehabilitation after head injury. *Br. med. J.,* **1**, 465–70

Lewin, W. (1970). Rehabilitation needs of the brain-injured patient. *Proc. R. Soc. Med.,* **63**, 28–32

Lindenberg, R., and Freytag, E. (1957). Morphology of cortical contusions. *Arch. Pathol.,* **63**, 23–42

Lindenberg, R , and Freytag, E. (1960). The mechanism of cerebral contu-sions. A pathologic-anatomic study. *Arch. Pathol.,* **69**, 440–69

Lishman, W. A. (1968). Brain damage in relation to psychiatric disability after head injury. *Br. J. Psychiat.,* **114**, 373–410

Lishman, W. A. (1973). The psychiatric sequelae of head injury: a review. *Psychol. Med.,* **3**, 304–18

Lissner, H. R., Gurdjian, E. S., and Webster, J. E. (1949). Mechanics of skull fracture. *Proc. Soc. exptl Stress Anal.,* **7**, 61–70

Logan, W. P. D., and Cushion, A. A. (1958). *Morbidity Statistics from General Practice,* Vol. I: *General.* London, HMSO

Logue, V., Durward, M., Pratt, R. T. C., Piercy, M., and Nixon, W. C. B. (1968). The quality of survival after rupture of an anterior cerebral aneurysm. *Br. J. Psychiat.*, **114**, 137–60

London, P. S. (1967). Some observations on the course of events after severe injury of the head. *Ann. R. Coll. Surgeons*, **41**, 460–79

Lundholm, A. J., Jepson, B., and Thornval, G. (1975a). Late sequelae of prolonged traumatic unconsciousness. Neurological, psychological and social aspects. *Ugeskrift Laeger*, **137**, 431–5

Lundholm, A. J., Jepson, B., and Thornval, G. (1975b). The late neurological, psychological and social aspects of severe traumatic coma. *Scand. J. Rehabil. Med.*, **7**, 97–100

McDowall, D. G., Barker, J., and Jennett, W. B. (1966). Cerebrospinal fluid pressure measurements during anaesthesia. *Anaesthesia*, **21**, 189–201

McFie, J. (1960). Psychological testing in clinical neurology. *J. nervous mental Dis.*, **131**, 383–93

Majumdar, S. K., and Bhushan, S. V. (1975). Hypopituitarism diagnosed long after head injury. *Practitioner*, **215**, 345–7

Maury, M., Audic, B., Lacombe, M., and Lucet, G. (1970). Re-education following head injuries. *Ann. Méd. phys.*, **13**, 47–58

Mealey, J. (1968). *Pediatric Head Injuries*. Springfield, Ill., Charles C. Thomas

Miller, E. (1970). Simple and choice reaction time following severe head injury. *Cortex*, **1**, 121–7

Miller, H. (1961a). Accident neurosis. Lecture 1. *Br. Med. J.*, **2**, 919–25

Miller, H. (1961b). Accident neurosis. Lecture 2. *Br. Med. J.*, **2**, 992–8

Miller, H. (1966). Mental after-effects of head injury. *Proc. R. Soc. Med.*, **59**, 257–61

Miller, H., and Stern, G. (1965). The long-term prognosis of severe head injury. *Lancet*, **i**, 225–9

Milner, B. (1969). Residual intellectual and memory deficits after head injury. In: Walker, A. E., Caveness, W. F., and Critchley, M. (eds), *The Late Effects of Head Injury*. Springfield, Ill., Charles C. Thomas, pp. 84–97

Miyasaki, K., Miyachi, Y., Arimitsu, K., Kita, E., and Yoshida, M. (1972). Post-traumatic hypothalamic obesity – an autopsy case. *Acta path. japon.*, **22**, 779–802

Narabayashi, H., and Uno, M. (1966). Long range results of stereotaxic amygdalotomy for behaviour disorders. *Confinia Neurol.*, **27**, 168–71

Narabayashi, H., Nagao, T., Saito, Y., Yoshida, M., and Nagahata, M. (1963). Stereotaxic amygdalotomy for behaviour disorders. *Arch. Neurol.*, **9**, 1–16

Nauta, W. J. H. (1964). Some efferent connections of the prefrontal cortex in the monkey. In: Warren, J. M., and Akert, K. (eds), *The Frontal Granular Cortex and Behavior*. New York, McGraw-Hill, pp. 397–409

Newcombe, F. (1969). *Missile Wounds of the Brain. A Study of Psychological Deficits*. Oxford, Oxford University Press

Nick, J., and Sicard-Nick, C. (1965). Les céphalées post-traumatiques tardives. Étude séméiologique, physiopathologique et thérapeutique. A propos de 240 cas. *Presse méd.*, **73**, 2587–92

Norrman, B., and Svahn, K. (1961). A follow-up study of severe brain injuries. *Acta psychiat. scand.*, **37**, 236–64

Obrador, S., Bustos, J. C., and Fernandez-Ruiz, L. C. (1973). Sequelae and functional reintegration following prolonged post-traumatic sub-reactivity. *Acta neurochir.*, **29**, 213–27

Okuma, T., Oda, T., and Matushita, T. (1973). A case of anterior pituitary insufficiency after head trauma. *Clin. Neurol.*, *Tokyo*, **13**, 506–12

Oldfield, R. C., and Wingfield, A. (1965). Response latencies in naming objects. *Q. Jl exp. Psychol.*, **17**, 273–81

Ommaya, A. K., and Gennarelli, T. A. (1974). Cerebral concussion and traumatic unconsciousness. Correlation of experimental and clinical observations on blunt head injuries. *Brain*, **97**, 633–54

Ommaya, A. K., Grubb, R. L., and Naumann, R. A. (1971). Coup and contre-coup injury: observations on the mechanics of visible brain injuries in the rhesus monkey. *J. Neurosurg.*, **35**, 503–16, 1971

Oppenheimer, D. R. (1968). Microscopic lesions in the brain following head injury. *J. Neurol. Neurosurg. Psychiat.*, **31**, 299–306

Ortegasuhrkamp, E., Faust, C., and Schulte, P. W. (1975). Late mental disorders and premature failure symptoms following brain injuries in middle-aged and elderly patients. *Aktuelle Gerontol.*, **5**, 405 ff.

Orthner, H., and Meyer, E. (1967). Der posttraumatische Diabetes insipidus. Befunde am neurosekretorischen System beim stumpfen Schädeltrauma, nebst Bemerkungen zum posttraumatischen Hirnödem. *Acta neurovegetat.*, *Wien*, **30**, 216–50

Overgaard, J., Hvid-Hansen, O., Land, M., Pederson, K. K. Christensen, S., Haase, J., Hein, O., Tweed, W. A. (1973). Prognosis after head injury based on early clinical examination. *Lancet*, **ii**, 631–5

Pagni, C. A. (1973). The prognosis of head injured patients in a state of coma with decerebrated posture: analysis of 471 cases. *J. neurosurg. Sci.*, **17**, 289–95

Panting, A., and Merry, P. H. (1972). The long-term rehabilitation of severe head injuries with particular reference to the need for social and medical support for the patient's family. *Rehabilitation*, **82**, 33–7

Papez, J. W. (1937). A proposed mechanism of emotion. *Arch. Neurol. Psychiat.*, *Chicago*, **38**, 725–43

Partridge, M. (1950). *Frontal Leucotomy*. Oxford, Blackwell

Payan, H., Toga, M., and Bérard–Badier, M. (1970). The pathology of post-traumatic epilepsies. *Epilepsia*, **11**, 81–94

Pazzaglia, P., Frank, G., Frank, F., and Gaist, G. (1975). Clinical course and prognosis of acute post-traumatic coma. *J. Neurol. Neurosurg. Psychiat.*, **38**, 149–54

Pedersen, K. K., and Haase, J. (1973). Isotope liquorgraphy in the demonstration of communicating obstructive hydrocephalus after severe cranial trauma. *Acta neurol. scand.*, **49**, 10–30

Penfield, W. (1927). The mechanism of cicatricial contraction in the brain. *Brain*, **50**, 499–517

Peserico, L., Merli, G. A., Gerosa, M., Galligioni, F., and Marin, G. (1973). Enlargement of the aqueduct of Sylvius as a complication of head injuries. *Neurochirurgia, Stuttgart*, **16**, 98–102

Piercy, M. (1964). The effects of cerebral lesions on intellectual function: a review of current research trends. *Br. J. Psychiat.*, **110**, 310–52

Plum, F., and Posner, J. B. (1972). *The Diagnosis of Stupor and Coma*, 2nd edn, Philadelphia, Davis

Polis, A. (1894). Experimental research into concussion. *Rev. Chirurgie*, **14**, 273–88

Porter, R. J., and Miller, R. A. (1948). Diabetes insipidus following closed head injury. *J. Neurol. Neurosurg. Psychiat.*, **11**, 258–62

Powell, T. P. S. (1973). Sensory convergence in the cerebral cortex. In: Laitinen, L. V. and Livingston, K. E. (eds). *Surgical Approaches in Psychiatry.* Lancaster, Medical & Technical Publishing Co. pp. 266–81

Pratt, R. T. C., and McKenzie, W. (1958). Anxiety states following vestibular disorders. *Lancet*, **ii**, 347–9

Price, D. J. E., and Murray, A. (1972). The influence of hypoxia and hypotension on recovery from head injury. *Injury*, **3**, 218–24

Rasmussen, T. (1969). Surgical therapy and posttraumatic epilepsy. In: Walker, A. E., Caveness, W. F., and Critchley, M. (eds). *The Late Effects of Head Injury.* Springfield, Ill., Charles C. Thomas, pp. 277–305

Raven, J. C. (1958). *Guide to the Standard Progressive Matrices and Extended Guide to Using the Mill Hill Vocabulary Scale with the Progressive Matrices.* London, H. K. Lewis

Registrar General's Statistical Review of England and Wales (1960). Part I. London, HMSO, 1962

Registrar General's Decennial Supplement. England and Wales (1961) Life Tables. London, HMSO, 1968

Reitmann, F. (1946). Orbital cortex syndrome following leucotomy. *Am. J. Psychiat.*, **103**, 238–41

Richardson, F. (1963). Some effects of severe head injury. A follow-up study of children and adolescents after protracted coma. *Devl Med. Child Neurol.*, **5**, 471–82

Roberts, A. H. (1964). Housebound housewives – a follow up study of a phobic anxiety state. *Br. J. Psychiat.*, **110**, 191–7

Roberts, A. H. (1969). *Brain Damage in Boxers. A Study of the Prevalence of Traumatic Encephalopathy among Ex-professional Boxers.* London, Pitman Medical

Robertson, R. C. L., and Pollard, C. (1968). Decerebrate state in children and adolescents. *J. Neurosurg.*, **12**, 13–17

Rodineau, J., Deseilligny, E. P., Bussel, B., and Held, J. P. (1970). Long-term motor prognosis in patients with severe cranial trauma. *Ann. Méd. phys.*, **13**, 25–32

Rowbotham, G. F. (1949). The long-term results of injuries of the head (a medical, economic and sociological survey). *J. mental Sci.*, **14**, 336–54

Rusk, H. A., Block, J. M., and Lowman, E. W. (1969). Rehabilitation of the brain-injured patient. A report of 157 cases with long-term follow-up of 118. In: Walker, A. E., Caveness, W. F. and Critchley, M. (eds), *The Late Effects of Head Injury.* Springfield, Ill., Charles C. Thomas, pp. 327–32

Russell, W. R. (1932). Cerebral involvement in head injury. A study based on the examination of two hundred cases. *Brain*, **55**, 549–603

Russell, W. R. (1933–4). The after-effects of head injury. *Trans. med. chir. Soc. Edinburgh*, **48**, 129–44 (New Series)

Russell, W. R. (1935). Amnesia following head injuries. *Lancet*, **ii**, 762–3

Russell, W. R. (1948–9). Traumatic amnesia. *Q. J. exptl Psychol.*, **1**, 2–6

Russell, W. R. (1966). Discussion, p. 266. In: Lishman, W. A.: Psychiatric disability after head injury: the significance of brain damage. *Proc. R. Soc. Med.*, **59**, 261–6

Russell, W. R., and Davies-Jones, G. A. B. (1969). Epilepsy following the brain wounds of World War II. In: Walker, A. E., Caveness, W. F., Critchley, M. (eds), *The Late Effects of Head Injury*. Springfield, Ill., Charles C. Thomas, pl. 189–92

Russell, W. R., and Nathan, P. W. (1946). Traumatic amnesia. *Brain*, **69**, 280–301

Russell, W. R., and Smith, A. (1961). Post traumatic amnesia in closed head injury. *Arch. Neurol.*, **5**, 4–17

Russell, W. R., and Whitty, C. W. M. (1952). Studies in traumatic epilepsy. 1. Factors influencing the incidence of epilepsy after brain wounds. *J. Neurol. Neurosurg. Psychiat.*, **15**, 93–8

Russell, R. G. G., Smith, R., Bishop, M. C., Price, D. A., and Squire, C. M. (1972). Treatment of myositis ossificans progressiva with a diphosphonate. *Lancet*, **i**, 10–12

Rylander, G. (1939). Personality changes after operations on the frontal lobes. *Acta Psychiat. Neurol.* Suppl 15

Sabauraut (1768). Sur les contre-coups dans les lesions de la tête. In: *Mémoires sur les sujets proposés pour les prix de l'Académie Royale de Chirurgie*, tome quatrième, premier partie. Chez Ménard et Desenne, Fils, Libraires, 1819, pp. 337–90

Salmon, J. H., and Timperman, A. L. (1971). Cerebral blood flow in posttraumatic encephalopathy. The effect of ventriculo-atrial shunt. *Neurology, Minn.*, **21**, 33–42

Sano, K., Yoshioka, M., Ogashiwa, M., Ishijima, B., and Ohye, C. (1966). Postero-medial hypothalamotomy in the treatment of aggressive behaviors. *Confinia neurol.*, **27**, 164–7

Sano, K., Ishijima, B., and Ohye, C. (1962). Sedative neurosurgery. *Neurol. med. chir., Tokyo*, **4**, 112 ff.

Sano, K., Nakamura, N., Hirakawa, K., Masuzawa, H., Hashizume, K., Hayashi, T., and Fujii, S. (1967). Mechanism and dynamics of closed head injury. *Neurol. med.-chir., Tokyo*, **9**, 21–3

Saucerotte (1769). Sur les contre-coups dans les lesions de la tête. In: *Mémoires sur les sujets proposés pour les prix de l'Académie Royale de Chirurgie*, tome quatrième, premier partie. Chez Ménard et Desenne, Fils, Libraires, 1819, pp. 290–337

Seddon, Sir H. (1972). *Surgical Disorders of the Peripheral Nerves.* Edinburgh and London, Churchill Livingstone

Sevitt, S. (1960). The significance and classification of fat-embolism. *Lancet*, **ii**, 825–8

Smith, E. (1974). Influence of site of impact on cognitive impairment persisting long after severe closed head injury. *J. Neurol. Neurosurg. Psychiat.*, **37**, 719–26

Sölch, O., and Schyra, B. (1972). The late results of severe cranio-cerebral injury. *Monats. Unfallheil.*, **75**, 141–55

Solé-Llenas, J., and Pons-Tortella, E. (1974). Ischaemic brain lesions associated with cerebral contusions. *Neurochirurgia*, **17**, 176–82

Spatz, H. (1950). Brain trauma in aviation. In: *German Aviation Medicine in World War II*. Surgeon General's Office, U.S. Air Force Department

Steele, J. C., Richardson, J. C., and Olszewski, J. (1964). Progressive supranuclear palsy. *Arch. Neurol.*, **10**, 333–59

Storey, P. B. (1967). Psychiatric sequelae of subarachnoid haemorrhage. *Br. med. J.*, **3**, 261–6

Strich, S. J. (1956). Diffuse degeneration of the cerebral white matter in severe dementia following head injury. *J. Neurol. Neurosurg. Psychiat.*, **19**, 163–85

Strich, S. J. (1961). Shearing of nerve fibres as a cause of brain damage due to head injury. A pathological study of twenty cases. *Lancet*, **ii**, 443–8

Strich, S. J. (1970). Lesions in the cerebral hemispheres after blunt head injury. *J. clin. Path.*, **23**, 166–71 (Suppl. 4)

Sunderland, Sir S. (1972). *Nerves and Nerve Injuries*. Edinburgh and London, Churchill Livingstone

Sweet, W. H., Ervin, F., and Mark, V. H. (1969). The relationship of violent behaviour to focal cerebral disease. In: Garattini, S., and Sigg, E. B. (eds), *Aggressive Behaviour*. Proceedings of the International Symposium on the Biology of Aggressive Behaviour, held in Milan, 2–4 May, 1968. Amsterdam, Excerpta Medica Foundation

Symonds, C. P. (1937). Mental disorder following head injury. *Proc. R. Soc. Med.*, **30**, 1081–94

Symonds, Sir C. (1962). Concussion and its sequelae. *Lancet*, **i**, 1–5

Szmeja, Z., Pruszewicz, A., Tokarz, F., Zwozdzia, K. W., and Obrebowski, A. (1974). Value of otoneurologic examinations in certification of late results of cranio-cerebral injuries. *Patologia Polska*, **25**, 469–73

Teasdale, G., and Jennett, B. (1974). Assessment of coma and impaired consciousness. A practical scale. *Lancet*, **ii**, 81–4

Terzian, G., and Dalle Ore, G. (1955). Syndrome of Klüver and Bucy reproduced in man by bilateral removal of the temporal lobes. *Neurology, Minn.*, **5**, 373–80

Teuber, H.-L. (1962). Effects of brain wounds implicating right and left hemisphere in man. In: Mountcastle, V. B. (ed.), *Interhemispheric Relations and Cerebral Dominance*. Baltimore, Johns Hopkins University Press

Teuber, H.-L. (1969). Neglected aspects of the posttraumatic syndrome. In: Walker, A. E., Caveness, W. F., and Critchley, M. (eds), *The Late Effects of Head Injury*. Springfield, Ill., Charles C. Thomas, pp. 13–34

Thorndyke, E. L., and Lorge, I. (1944). *The Teacher's Word Book of 30,000 Words*. New York, Teachers' College, Columbia University

Toglia, J. U., Rosenberg, P. E., and Ronis, M. L. (1970). Posttraumatic dizziness. Vestibular, audiologic and medicolegal aspects. *Arch. Otolaryngol.*, **92**, 485–92

Tomlinson, B. E. (1970). Brain stem lesions after head injury. *J. clin. Path.*, **23**, 154–65 (Suppl. 4)

Treip, C. S. (1970). Hypothalamic and pituitary injury. *J. clin. Path.*, **23**, 178–86 (Suppl. 4)

Tubbs, O. N., and Potter, J. M. (1970). Early post concussional headache. *Lancet*, **ii**, 128–9

Turner, J. W. A. (1943). Indirect injuries of the optic nerve. *Brain*, **66**, 140–51

van der Zwan, A. (1969). Late results from prolonged traumatic unconsciousness. In: Walker, A. E., Caveness, W. F., and Critchley, M. (eds), *The Late Effects of Head Injury*. Springfield, Ill., Charles C. Thomas, pp. 138–41

Vapalahti, M., and Troupp, H. (1971). Prognosis for patients with severe brain injuries. *Br. med. J.*, **3**, 404–7

Vigouroux, P. R., Baurand, C., Choux, M., and Guillermain, P. (1972). État actuel des aspects séquellaires graves dans les traumatismes craniens de l'adulte. *Neurochirurgie*, **18**, (Suppl. 2)

Walker, A. E., and Erculei, F. (1969). *Head Injured Men Fifteen Years Later*. Springfield, Ill., Charles C. Thomas

Walker, A. E., and Erculei, F. (1970). Post traumatic epilepsy 15 years later. *Epilepsia, Amsterdam*, **11**, 17–26

Walker, A. E., and Jablon, S. (1961). *A Follow-up Study of Head Wounds in World War II*. Washington D.C., Veterans Administration Medical Monograph, U.S. Government Printing Office

Walker, A. E., Leuchs, H. K., Lechtape-Grüter, H., Caveness, W. R., and Kretschman, C. (1971). Life expectancy of head injured men with and without epilepsy. *Arch. Neurol.*, **24**, 95–100

Walsh, F. B., and Hoyt, W. F. (1969). *Clinical Neuro-ophthalmology*, Vol. 3: *Craniocerebral Trauma, Hypoxia, and Injuries by other Physical Agents: Involvement of the Visual and Ocular Motor System*. Baltimore, Williams & Wilkins, pp. 2331–518

Wechsler, D. (1944). *The Measurement of Adult Intelligence*, 3rd edn, Baltimore, Williams & Wilkins

Wechsler, D. (1945). A standardised memory scale for clinical use. *J. Psychol.*, **19**, 87–95

Willoughby, J. O., and Leach, B. G. (1974). Relation of neurological findings after cardiac arrest to outcome. *Br. med. J.*, **3**, 437–9

Wolff, H. G. (1963). *Headache and Other Pain*, 2nd edn, New York, Oxford University Press

Woolf, P. D., and Schalch, D. S. (1973). Hypopituitarism secondary to hypothalamic insufficiency. *Ann. intern. Med.*, **78**, 88–90

Wowern, F. von (1966). Obesity as a sequel of traumatic injury to the hypothalamus. *Danish med. Bull.*, **13**, 11–13

Zangwill, O. L. (1960). *Cerebral Dominance and its Relation to Psychological Function*. Edinburgh, Oliver & Boyd

Zieman, W., and King, F. A. (1958). Tumours of the septum pellucidum and adjacent structures with abnormal affective behaviour: an anterior midline structure syndrome. *J. nervous mental Dis.*, **127**, 490–502

Zülch, K.-L. (1969). Medical causation. In: Walker, A. E., Caveness, W. F., and Critchley, M. (eds), *The Late Effects of Head Injury*. Springfield, Ill. Charles C. Thomas, pp. 453–72

Index

Accident, type of 37, 39
Age (*see also* Children)
   and anosmia 90, 100
   and facial palsy 95, 100
   at injury 30–1
   and neurohypophyseal damage
     105–6
   in predicting outcome 152–79,
     184–5
   previous reports 5–17, 19
   and progressive encephalopathy
     130–3, 137
   and psychometric test results
     67–74
Ageing, premature 129–39, 184
Agoraphobia 60, 62, 84
Akinesia *see* Slowness
Akinetic mutism 47
Alzheimer's disease 134, 136–9
Anosmia 5–7, 11, 89–90, 182
   and age 90, 100
   and coal-gas poisoning 93
Anxiety 6, 14, 57, 60–2, 81,
   83–4
   phobic, and imbalance 60,
   84
Apallic state *see* Vegetative and
   analogous states
Ataxia, cerebellar 5, 6, 7, 11, 13,
   15–16, 40
   see also Neural disability, central
   (physical), brainstem cerebellar
Athetosis 41
   see also Neural disability, central
   (physical), athetoid pseudobulbar

Boxers' encephalopathy 2, 78–9,
   82–3, 129, 138

Brachial plexus 5, 113
Brain
   compression 29, 79–81
   distribution of damage
     in mental disability 56–62,
     77–83, 86–8
     in neurophysical disability
     39–54
   penetration
     accidental 29
     and epilepsy 118–28
     missile 1–2, 83
     surgical 29
   swelling 42, 50–2
Bulimia *see* Hyperphagia

Children 6, 8, 15–17, 152–79
Choice reaction time task 87–8
Cingulate gyric and intracranial
   pressure necrosis 79–81
Cognitive function
   see Psychometric tests
Coma
   as criterion of severity of injury
     4–10, 13, 33–5
   definition of 30, 37
   duration of, predicting outcome
     8–17, 155–8
   and epilepsy 118, 120, 126
   grade of, predicting outcome
     17–18
   previous reports 8–18
   and psychometric tests 67, 71,
     87
   work capacity, relation to 8–10
Compensation 25–6, 84
Concentration, impairment of 5, 9
Contre-coup brain injury 43, 45,
   50, 52–4
   in boxers 2

and dysphasia   86
and electroencephalogram   53, 125
and occupational status   76
and psychometric tests   66–7, 86–7
Corpus callosum   53–4
Cranial nerve lesions   5–7, 11, 89–96, 100–1, 182–3
    see also Anosmia, Deafness, Facial palsy, Oculomotor palsies, Optic nerve lesions, Trigeminal nerves and Vertigo and vestibular disorders

Deafness   7, 11, 89, 96, 183
Death, causes of   140–51
    compared with general population   147–50
    epilepsy   118, 127
    progressive dementia   135–7
Decerebrate response
    definition   30, 37–8
    instantaneous   50
    as measure of severity of injury   33–5
    and neurohypophyseal damage   105–6
    as predictor of outcome   12, 15–20, 152–79
    and psychometric test results   67–71, 87
    see also Neural disability, central (physical), decerebrate dementia
Dementia   5–11, 55–9, 63–6, 77–88
    as cause of death   135–7, 148
    progressive   129–39
Depressive illness   6, 11, 14, 57, 61, 63, 66, 205–6
Diabetes insipidus   102–7, 109

Disability, definition of grades of   177–9
    central neural   40
    mental   56
Disequilibrium   39, 51
Disinhibition   14, 55, 57
Drowning   143, 147–8
Dysarthria   5, 11, 16, 39
Dysphasia   5–7, 10, 11, 62
    and side of head impact   46, 86

Electroencephalogram
    and contre-coup brain injury   53, 125
    and focal epilepsy   124–5
Employment   see Work capacity
Endocrine disfunction   7, 102–10, 183
Enuresis   107–8
Epidemiological implications   186–90
Epilepsy   118–28, 184
    as cause of death   118, 127, 143–7, 149–50, 184
    and paranoid psychosis   63–5
    previous reports   6, 9, 11, 13
Euphoria   8, 55, 57

Facial palsy   5–7, 11, 92, 95, 100, 183
Fat emboli   115, 117
Fornices   62
Fractures
    of limbs   113–17
    of skull   36
        and anosmia   89–90
        and facial palsy   92, 95, 183
        and optic nerve lesions   90, 93
        and prolonged coma   52
        and side of head impact   43, 45
Frontal lobes   see Mental disorders and disabilities

Haematoma, extradural and
        subdural   29, 35, 78–81
    and epilepsy   118–28
Headache   98–101, 183
Hippocampal gyri   79–81
Hydrocephalus   135, 138–9
Hygroma   35
Hyperkinesia   16, 57
Hyperphagia   102–10, 183
Hypoplasia of limbs   17, 202
Hypothalamus
    disconnection of   80–1
    disorders of   102–10, 183

Imbalance   see Disequilibrium
Impotence   103–4, 107, 109
    and pathological jealousy   63
Incoordination   see Ataxia,
        cerebellar
Infarction   41, 42, 50–2, 60, 116,
        155, 180
    brain, and shear strain damage
        50, 60, 180
    brainstem   50
Intellectual functions
    impairment   5–16, 55–88
    tests   see Mental disorders and
        disabilities and Psychometric
        tests
Intracranial pressure, raised   9, 20,
        50, 79–81
Irritability   5, 9, 13, 14, 16,
        55–62, 77–83
    and hypothalamic injury   110,
        183

Jealousy, pathological   63

Leucotomies, frontal, effects of   8,
        57, 60, 107
Libido   102–4, 107, 109

and frontal lobe damage   77
and pathological jealousy   63
and temporal lobe damage   77
Life expectancy   6, 135–7,
        140–51
    in decerebrate dementia
        140–3, 151
    in those discharged from
        hospital   142–50
    in progressive dementia   135–7
    in those remaining in hospital
        140–2, 150–1
Limbic lobes   56–7, 82

Mamillary bodies   62
Memory impairment   7, 9, 10,
        55–88
    and anxiety   60–2
    in boxers   78–80
    progressive   134–8
    and shear strain damage   77–81
    and side of head impact   66
    and slow mentation   88
    in steeplechase jockeys   83
Meningitis   112, 116
    as cause of death   143–8
Mental disorders and disabilities
        55–88
    grades of   55
    paranoid delusional illness
        62–5, 85, 129–34, 182
    patterns of
        dysmnesic inadequacy   61–2,
            83–4, 182, 203–5
        frontal   60, 200–1
        frontal dysmnesia   60, 182
        frontal irritable   62, 110, 183
        frontolimbic dementia
            57–60, 181–2, 194–9
        irritability and forgetfulness
            57–60
        phobic imbalance   60–1,
            83–4, 182

Mental disorders—*cont.*
  traumatic dysmnesia   62,
    82–3, 182, 199–203
  previous reports   5–10
  schizophreniform psychosis
    63–5, 85, 129–34, 182
  scores   55
Microglial clusters   53–4
Missile injury   1–2, 83, 86
  and epilepsy   126–7, 184
Mortality rate   *see* Life expectancy
Motor response to stimulation
  deterioration in level of, in
    patterns of residual neural
    disability   49–54
  as indicator of deterioration due
    to cerebral infarction
    42–3
  as predictor of outcome   19–20,
    152–79, 184–5
  and psychometric tests   67–74,
    86–7
Myositis ossificans   115–17

Neural disability, central (physical)
  athetoid pseudobulbar   41–3,
    48–54, 194–6
    life expectancy in   141–2
    mental disorder in   57
  brainstem cerebellar   41–2,
    49–54, 197–201
    life expectancy in   41–2
    mental disorder in   57
  decerebrate dementia   41,
    47–54, 191–4
    life expectancy in   41, 140–2,
    150–1, 180–1, 189
  grades of   39–40
  hemiparetic   41–2, 49–54,
    201–4
    and side of head impact   43,
    45, 50, 52–4
  patterns of   39–54, 130–3,
    137–8, 180–2, 191–4

  degrees of disability in   44
  previous reports   5–17
  progressive encephalopathy
    130–3, 137–8
  scores   40
  see also Mental disorders

Obesity   7, 11, 109–10
Obsessional symptomatology   66,
  88
Occupation   *see* Work capacity
Oculomotor palsies   5, 6, 11, 17,
  89, 91, 94–5, 100, 183
Optic nerve lesions   5–7, 11, 90,
  93–4, 100–1, 183
  and neurohypophyseal injury
    108
Outcome   *see* Disability, definition
  of grades of

Paranoid dementia   5, 62–5,
  129–34, 182
Pareses, limbs
  minor hemiparesis   14, 41–2,
    49
  previous reports   5–17
  severe hemiparesis   42
  and side of head impact   50,
    52–4
  see also Neural disability, central
    (physical), hemiparetic
Parkinson's disease   11, 14,
  136–7
Pathology   41–3, 49–54, 77–81,
  180
  epilepsy   127–8
  hypothalamus   102, 110
  optic nerves   101
  progressive encephalopathy
    136–8
Peripheral nerve injury   113
Personality change   55–66,
  75–85

frontal   57−62, 77, 80−1
improvement   5, 57, 60, 81
previous reports   5−10, 13−14
progressive decerebration
    129−39
and side of head impact   66
Phobic imbalance   60−2, 83−4
Pituitary hypofunction   102−10,
    183
Post-concussional state   5, 84, 87
Post-traumatic amnesia (PTA)
  and anosmia   89−90
  as criterion of severity of injury
    33−5
  and death among those
    discharged from hospital
    143−8
  definition   30
  and epilepsy   118, 120, 126
  and neurohypophyseal damage
    105−6
  and optic, external ocular and
    facial nerve lesions   90−2
  and patterns of mental
    disability   60−1
  and prediction   159−79, 184−5
  previous reports   5−6, 9−10, 13
  and progressive
    encephalopathy   130−3,
    137
  and psychometric tests   67−74,
    87
  and vertigo   97
Prediction of outcome   152−79,
    184−5
  incorrect   167−73
  and occupation   174−6
  prolonged coma and   155−8
  PTA and   159−79
  rate of recovery and   152−9,
    161−3
  summary   173−4
  worst state of neurological
    dysfunction and   159−79
Progressive encephalopathy

129−39, 183−4
Psychiatric disabilities   55−88,
    110, 182−3
  previous reports   5−17
Psychometric tests   27, 66−74,
    85−7
  and mental disability   72−6,
    86−7
  previous reports   16, 86−7
  and PTA   67−74, 87
  and severity of injury   67−74,
    86−7

Recovery, rate of
  in haematoma   154−5
  in prediction of outcome
    152−9, 161−3
  previous reports, 6, 8, 16

Satiety centres and hyperphagia
    103−10
Schizophrenia, schizophreniform
    psychosis   5, 11, 63−5, 85,
    129−34, 182
Sensory deficits, cortical   5−7, 10,
    14, 43, 45
Sexual function   see Libido
Shear strain brain injury   50,
    53−4, 57, 60, 77−80, 81, 83,
    180
Slowness
  of movement   17, 41, 51
  of speech   7
  of thought   7, 9, 14, 17, 87−8
Smell, sense of   see Anosmia
Spasticity, recovery of   5−6, 8,
    15−16, 51
Suicide   14, 66, 85, 143−8, 182

Temporal lobes
  contusions   80
  epilepsy   124−5, 128

Temporal lobes—*cont.*
  and hippocampal and medial
    pressure necrosis   79–81,
    83–4
  and periamygdaloid areas and
    rage   82
  and site of head impact   53, 87
  and slowness of movement and
    thought   88
Trigeminal nerves   95, 183

Unconsciousness   *see* Coma

Vegetative and analogous states

    10, 20, 47–8, 50
  experimental models of   88
  survival in   10, 47, 140–2,
    150–1, 180–1, 189
Vertigo and vestibular disorders
    11, 96–8, 101, 183
  adrenalin loading   84
  and drowning   147–8
Visual field defects   90, 93–4,
    100–1
  homonymous cortical   11, 17,
    43, 45

Work capacity   74–6, 182
  previous reports   6–10, 13